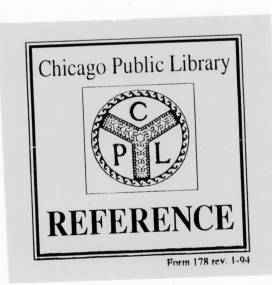

THE POWER OF
PERIMENOPAUSE

THE POWER OF PERIMENOPAUSE

A Woman's Guide to Physical and Emotional Health During the Transitional Decade

BY

STEPHANIE DeGRAFF BENDER

WITH TREACY COLBERT

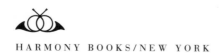

HARMONY BOOKS/NEW YORK

Published by Harmony Books, a division of Crown Publishers, Inc., 201 East 50th Street, New York, New York 10022. Member of the Crown Publishing Group.

Random House, Inc. New York, Toronto, London, Sydney, Auckland
www.randomhouse.com

HARMONY and colophon are trademarks of Crown Publishers, Inc.

Printed in the United States of America

Design by June Bennett-Tantillo

Library of Congress Cataloging-in-Publication Data

Bender, Stephanie DeGraff.
    The power of perimenopause: a woman's guide to physical and emotional health during the transitional decade / by Stephanie DeGraff Bender, with Treacy Colbert.—1st ed.
        p.   cm.
    1. Menopause—Popular works.   2. Middle aged women—Health and hygiene.   3. Middle aged women—Psychology.   I. Colbert, Treacy.   II. Title.
RG186.B464   1998
618.1'75—dc21   97-40595
                                            CIP

ISBN 0-517-70894-9

10 9 8 7 6 5 4 3 2 1

First Edition

Lovingly dedicated to my sons, Billy and Tim, and to my husband, Bill. It has enriched my forties decade to have spent them with the three of you. Also dedicated in loving memory to Suzanne Lipsett.

ACKNOWLEDGMENTS

I would like to thank all of the women — and there have been more than ten thousand of you over nearly two decades — who have allowed me the privilege of knowing you and your unique circumstances. This book would not have been possible without your generosity of spirit. I am also deeply grateful to Marla Ahlgrimm, R.Ph., Candice Fuhrman, Nancy Adams, Jim Bender, Stephen O. James, John Kells, Scott Cloud, Rowena Stout, Leslie Meredith, Laura Wood, Terri Pobanz, Peter M. Greenly, Monica Martin, Bob Laemle, Mary Elizabeth Bissell M.D., and Molly Romary M.D. Special thanks to Treacy Colbert, who helped me make this book possible with her invaluable editorial insight, sense of humor, and steadfastness in the face of every challenge.

CONTENTS

CHAPTER ONE

Perimenopause:
The Big Picture

I'm often invited to speak on issues of hormonal health to groups of women in their forties. Looking out over the audience, I see an amazing diversity among the women — some are still girlish, some are distinctly mature; some are fashionably slender, some are rounding out; some look energetic and alert, some a little tired. But what I can't tell by looking is who is a grandmother, who a first-time mother of a preschooler, who a single woman over the span of adult life, who a divorced or widowed woman newly entering the category of "single woman." Who of these women has chosen to pass up childbearing and remain "child free"? Who has been struggling for decades with infertility and is now considering adoption, and who is taking advantage of the innovative options for conception yielded by a virtually exploding technology? Who is in a stable, long-term relationship, and who is — for want of a better word — dating?

Such an audience, in all its diversity, is a perfect symbol for the subject of this book: the forties, the transitional decade in a woman's life. It's the diversity itself that makes my audience a perfect symbol, because although the decade is marked by changes as distinct as those between ages 10 and 20, each woman goes through them at her own pace and with her own physiological and hormonal "style." The *changes* are the same, but the ways of undergoing them, and to some extent the time it takes to do so, are related to the individual.

The random person on the street, be it a woman or a man, wouldn't necessarily agree that individual styles evolve within this decade of change. That's because, in our youth-oriented culture, the forties have a bad reputation: too often they're viewed as the last, desperate period of a woman's real life before *the end*—menopause, that is—after which old age sets in with a vengeance. This stereotype is pervasive; I often hear it expressed by clients when they first come to my women's health clinic, Full Circle. All too often they feel they're headed toward a fall, speeding toward the cliff that will mark the end of their lives as attractive, productive, sexual women—so much so that they interpret the various changes they experience in body and psyche only as dreaded signals that they are fast approaching "the change." The true nature of the forties decade—its physical, intellectual, and emotional qualities—are an indistinct blur, like the terrain outside the window of a supersonic train. My goal at my clinic, and in writing this book, is to shatter the "end of life" stereotype, to explain the particular processes and changes that characterize the forties, and to slow down the train.

The "last chance" stereotype persists for a good reason: we have too little information to the contrary. Even many of the most supportive books on menopause focus on it as if it suddenly *happened* sometime at the end of the forties or the beginning of the fifties, as if it were an *event* unrelated to anything that came before. In fact, although menopause is indeed a milestone on a woman's developmental path, it is also a link in a long chain of events—physiological and psychological—that precede it. To a greater or lesser degree, we experience these events as changes, and sometimes as distressing symptoms, in our bodies, our emotions, our sexuality, and in other areas of our lives. To a greater or lesser degree, the medical world has tended to brush aside these changes as "just signs of aging," developments not worth treating and to which we women might as well just become accustomed. For this reason, most women get neither the information they need to understand what's happening to them nor the advice or treatment—often pretty minimal—that could ease any discomfort they might experience.

There's one more reason that the forties decade has remained in the shadows for us — and I say "us" accurately, for I am 47 as I write this. We women in our forties now are baby boomers, and during our teenage years our mothers were 1950s "ladies," strapped by the conventions and conformities of that particularly stringent decade. In an effort to prevent all the "terrible symptoms" associated with menopause from developing, many of our mothers underwent hysterectomies *before* they plummeted off that cliff. Others followed the rules by simply not speaking of the "change of life," and their silence added an aura of ominous gloom to the subject. So most of us have no role models for adapting to the changes in the transition decade with interest, initiative, and a commitment to self-care.

It is my aim, both in my clinic and in this book, to change all that by filling in the information gap. This book shines a beam of light onto the forties decade for women and fully explains the developments that occur in both the physical and psychological realms. Handily enough, although medical science has generally ignored the forties as vague and uninteresting, it has given a name to this portion of the developmental arc. That name is *perimenopause,* and the goal of my work as a medical caregiver and educator is to make that term as familiar to the general public as *menopause* is today.

The prefix *peri* literally means "that which surrounds," but the word *perimenopause* is used to refer to the events leading up to menopause. For some women, perimenopause lasts less than a decade; for others, it is somewhat longer. Individuals experience perimenopause differently, just as they do the transition into fertility during puberty. Still, for most women, the period of perimenopause roughly corresponds to the years from 40 to 50, and for those who fall outside that decade, the changes are the same.

A PROFILE OF OUR CHANGES

The purpose of this chapter is to sketch the big picture: what happens during the perimenopausal period, and therefore how we differ at age 40 from age 50. In subsequent chapters, I will return to each of these changes and focus on it in detail. Here I want to describe a certain kind of woman whom I meet time and time again at my lectures and seminars on perimenopause and women's hormonal health. After my talk, she will come up to me with an excited smile on her face. "Everything you said applies to me!" she'll exclaim. "Have you been following me around my house? I can't believe it. You described me to a T!"

She is in her midforties and is committed to learning all she can about her own health. She has come to my lecture, probably with a friend, because she has a number of questions about changes she's been experiencing in her body, changes that her ob/gyn has waved away as unimportant. I'll let her express these concerns in her own voice, then in addressing them, I'll sketch an overview of the major events of perimenopause.

"*I used to have periods as regular as clockwork, but they're different now. What's happening?*" The reproductive years form a kind of spectrum within the wider developmental phases of a woman's life. They begin at about age 12, at menarche, which means the beginning of menstruation. The biological plan — which conflicts with customs surrounding reproduction in most Western cultures, including our own — seems to be that a girl begins procreating as soon as she is physically and psychologically strong enough to show some independence.

One's first menstrual period is a landmark event — for most women, the memory of the experience is indelible. But like all biological occurrences, that first period is just one link in a chain of complex interactions and processes that take place over the prepubescent years. For several years before menstruation actually begins, a girl's ovaries begin to produce estrogen in response to another hormone, called follicle-stimulating hormone (FSH); its release is stimulated by the hypothalamus, a part of the brain. As with menarche, so with menopause: both are only the most noticeable in a complex series of interrelated processes.

What follows menarche is a period of thirty to thirty-five years — the fully fertile, reproductive years — in which each month the ovaries make available for fertilization one of the many eggs within them. Another function of the ovaries is to produce the primary female hormones, or chemicals that regulate various physiological and psychological processes. By the time we reach our forties, our ovaries are in the process of winding down their production of hormones, thereby slowly, *gradually* causing our reproductive potential to taper off.

Picture women's fertility, then, as a gentle arc, gradually prepared for, strongly functioning over about a thirty-five-year period, and gradually tapering off. During the tapering-off time, the perimenopausal decade, our ovaries' production of the primary female hormones, estrogen and progesterone, fluctuates. Those fluctuations, in turn, create some noticeable physical changes, one of which is changes in the menstrual cycle.

During your fully fertile years, you may have had a highly regular cycle, with a menstrual period beginning every twenty-eight days. Now, however, somewhere in your forties, you may be having a period every twenty-four to twenty-five days, and the period itself may be different. Have you gone from what was to you a normal four-to-five-day flow to a scanty one-to-two-day flow? Or have you, for example, had shorter cycles for a while, followed by a skipped period every now and then, followed by a series of periods separated by thirty-eight or forty days? Do you, perhaps, experience more cramping now than you did before?

Such irregularities send lots of women flying to their gynecologists in alarm. "Does all of this mean that something is wrong? What's going on?" Most often they get a resounding no! in response to the first question — definitely the correct answer — but they get no answer at all to the second.

What's going on is that the hormonal balance in your body is shifting. During the years of full fertility, estrogen causes the uterine lining (the endometrium) to thicken, and that material is later sloughed off as menstrual flow. But when estrogen production declines, less lining builds up, which means there is less tissue to be sloughed off.

"I feel depressed sometimes for no reason. I used to get blue around my periods, and this feels the same, but I can't figure out whether there's a connection." Changes in your menstrual flow or in the way you feel around the time of menstruation all have to do with the decline in your hormonal production. Perhaps one of the most disconcerting effects is that the changes in your cycle make it harder to predict your moods. Ask most women in their fully fertile years whether they like having a men-

strual period every month, and most will probably answer "No way!" Yet for others a regular period serves as a marker, an event that carries with it—and serves to explain—unpleasant symptoms such as depression, "mood swings," physical bloating, or food cravings. These symptoms might worry a woman, had she not experienced them for a decade or two in conjunction with her periods. In the twenties and thirties, this regularity goes a long way toward relieving women's anxiety around those symptoms, but in perimenopause we find ourselves a little more at sea.

"I'm waking up in the middle of the night drenched in sweat, and during the day I have hot flashes. Does this mean that I'm in menopause? Aren't I too young for that? And besides, I'm still having periods." As estrogen levels go down during perimenopause, levels of FSH are going up. The function of FSH is to cause a follicle to grow in the ovary, and during perimenopause it is still trying to get the ovary to produce one more egg each month in a kind of last hurrah. One of the side effects of FSH is to dilate the blood vessels that lie directly under the skin. Blood rushes into the dilated blood vessels, causing a sudden sensation of warmth or heat. During sleep, some women experience this rush of blood to the surface as night sweats.

Whenever we experience a hot flash, the first thing any of us think is, "Menopause!" If we're in our early forties, that thought is followed by the inevitable, "But I'm way too young to be experiencing that!" The fact is, though, that about 85 percent of women in their perimenopausal years experience hot flashes or night sweats. For some, it will not be a problem; others will be uncomfortable enough to seek medical help. Both self-treatments and medical interventions are available that can ease hormonally induced internal temperature disturbances, and I will discuss these later in the book.

"I've never had any trouble sleeping, but now all of a sudden I'm wrestling with insomnia." Insomnia is second only to hot flashes as the most noticeable physical symptom of perimenopause, and it frequently motivates women to seek help. Few women actually connect their new sleep problems with hormonal changes, but perimenopausal changes can actually interfere with sleep in a number of ways. Night sweats—the hot flashes that occur during sleep—can wake us up, even from a deep

sleep. If you wake up in the night to find your nightgown drenched, you may have difficulty going back to sleep. But other patterns of insomnia interfere more directly with sleep: for example, some women have trouble getting to sleep at all, while others have difficulty staying asleep.

Sleep disorders are among our great unsolved mysteries. In fact, sleep itself—the reason for it—has puzzled scientists throughout the ages and continues to do so. They still can't answer the seemingly basic, straightforward question, "Why do we need to sleep?" Recent research, however, has suggested that sleep interferences may have to do with the interrelationships between hormones and a neurotransmitter called serotonin. Neurotransmitters are chemicals produced by our bodies that, among other things, affect our sleep patterns and moods. Recent discoveries suggest that neurotransmitters and hormones may be strongly linked to each other. Although the picture is as yet very sketchy, it is possible that the decrease in female hormones during perimenopause affects the levels of serotonin, resulting in interferences with sleep.

Whatever their causes, however, we know that sleep interruptions can have negative effects on many aspects of our lives. Insomnia can cause not only physical but emotional fatigue, and it can threaten our overall sense of well-being. As with all the effects of perimenopause, there are many ways to control insomnia. (I'll describe them in chapter 4.) But the first step to reducing the disruptions that insomnia can cause is to realize that insomnia can have many causes and that it comes about as part of the process natural to the forties. No, you're not anxious about something you haven't yet identified. No, you haven't necessarily overstressed yourself without knowing it. No, you don't have to live with this and just get used to it because it's your "time of life." Yes, it is part of perimenopause. It's natural, explainable—and treatable.

"All of a sudden I don't recognize my body. I know I haven't been eating more, but my waist is gone, and everything seems to be going to my bottom. I don't think I'm fatter, but the sands are definitely shifting." There's no getting around it: in our forties we come up against some definite stumbling blocks when it comes to projecting that hourglass figure. (Did anyone really have it, ever?) Not only is our hormone production slowing, but so is our metabolism, which means we need fewer calories to maintain our body weight. At the same time, another hormone comes

into more active play: thyroid. This chemical is involved in the metabolism of food, and it is very difficult to track.

These factors lead to shifts in body shape and the increased production of fatty tissue. It's not the most welcome news, I know. Yet there's a rationale behind our increased fat production: as our ovaries reduce their estrogen production, the fat cells take over the job of synthesizing the hormone. In this way they safeguard the body against being completely devoid of estrogen during the perimenopausal years.

Another part of the fat-cell picture has to do with changes in our breast tissue. Because estrogen stimulates breast tissue, it stands to reason that when estrogen levels drop, breast tissue changes too. The effect is fattier, less firm breast tissue that causes breasts to seem less elastic and often to give way more to gravity. The tissue is less dense as well, which makes breasts easier to examine during years when the risk of breast cancer increases. That's one advantage, anyway.

"I've always been proud of my complexion, but now my skin looks terrible." Skin gains its elasticity from a substance called collagen. When estrogen levels drop, collagen production slows, and often the skin begins to wrinkle. For some women, the changes are hardly noticeable; for others, they are more obvious. Many of the women who come to my clinic are mourning the loss of their peaches-and-cream look. I suggest to them that they treat themselves to a facial, turning a necessity into a luxurious, sensual experience while restoring oils to a drying skin.

"Sex has always been important to me, but nowadays it's so uncomfortable, I'm starting to get turned off. Is it true, after all, that after forty women just aren't very sexual?" Not at all. We've all heard the cliché that our minds are our most important erogenous zone, and that doesn't change with age. What does happen during perimenopause, as a result of the decrease in estrogen, is a thinning and drying of the vaginal tissues. The result can be discomfort—often a great deal of discomfort—during sex, resulting in a distinct loss of responsiveness. But there are a whole range of measures that can be taken to help, some as simple as using a sexual lubricant. In fact, sexual activity can actually be more enjoyable during perimenopause than before—with a little attention to the issue in question.

"I think I must have an early case of Alzheimer's disease. I just can't concentrate on anything." For many women, the forties are a time when their life circumstances finally allow them to focus more completely on work. It can be very distressing, then, when absentmindedness, confusion, and an inability to concentrate make their appearance. But actually the causes of these symptoms may be relatively easy to identify and remedy. Diet may well be a cause: perhaps you are eating sporadically, or eating a sugar-based diet that causes your blood sugar level to fluctuate and keeps you in a fog. Or perhaps you need to be exercising more to increase your alertness and keep your blood sugar level even, with no sudden dips. Maybe you are inducing "adrenaline rushes" in yourself by overindulging in sugar, caffeine, or alcohol. A decrease in estrogen can also interfere with your ability to remain mentally alert. For women in their twenties and thirties, the latter problem would not come up, but for perimenopausal women it has great relevance, and addressing it may turn out to be the simple solution to a serious, anxiety-producing problem.

Many, many other questions arise in my clinic sessions with women in their forties — concerns about shifting interests, nutritional matters, energy levels, mood swings . . . the list goes on and on. Generally, I schedule three one-hour sessions to talk to such women about perimenopause and zero in on their hormonal health concerns, but recently a woman named Gloria came in to see me who could not afford the cost of the full three hours. She was a 45-year-old ex-athlete — a former professional tennis player — who had retired to have children. Now her daughter was six and her son four.

We had already met once, and she had called to ask if I could squeeze the rest of my workup into just one more hourlong meeting, instead of two more. I agreed, but reluctantly. I had recently returned from a lecture in which I talked for three and a half hours on the subject of women's hormonal health to a lay audience. How on earth, I wondered, was I going to squeeze the ever-growing list of perimenopause-related concerns, to which patients add new issues and questions every day, into a single hour? But my efforts to meet the challenge paid off, for my preparations for Gloria's visit crystallized my thinking on perimenopause as a whole. I realized that perimenopause is not just a phase of a woman's life; it represents a shift in a woman's consciousness, away from an old and distorting point of view about life.

When Gloria came in to talk to me, everything about her expressed exasperation. "I'm just going crazy!" she cried. "When is all of this going to stop? I finally got my kids sleeping in their own beds. I finally have both kids in school a major part of the day. I finally got to where I could take a part-time job and get out of the house once in a while. I finally gained control of my diet so that I've lost most of the weight I gained during pregnancy. I finally found the right moisturizing cream for my skin, and on and on. But now I'm being absolutely plagued with insomnia. I go to sleep, and two hours later I wake up. And that's it for the rest of the night. Maybe I fall into a doze, but I just can't get any real sleep. As a result, I'm irritated with my children, cranky with my husband, and sullen beyond belief at work. I'm asking you, Stephanie, when is all of this going to end? When can I expect to be *finished* with all this and get on with my *life*?"

Ah! I thought. That's the heart of the distortion exactly. Finished? But we're never finished changing, growing, moving at a steady pace toward maturity. Change *is* life; we change until we die. Physical and psychological processes continue to change even elderly people for specific reasons directly related to their phase of life. Until very recently, however, the fact that adults change and develop was a radical idea to people: "'The development of adults'? I don't understand. It's children who develop. Once you've grown up, well—that's it, right?"

Not at all. "Let me put it this way," I said to Gloria. "I'm afraid that the short answer to 'when is this going to end?' is never, or at least that the changes will go on as long as you are alive. But expecting to finally be finished somehow, all grown up and ready to go out into the world, is the result of seeing things in a distorted way. Think about your kids, for instance. You've never had any trouble relating certain characteristics and problems that they might have to their ages, right? I mean, kids under one year old often have ear infections, grammar-school kids who have difficulty reading often have social problems, kids entering adolescence frequently have trouble in school. Not only do you recognize certain problems as age-related, but making that connection helps you to understand the problems, right?"

Gloria nodded. "Yes, of course."

"Well, I want to suggest that you widen that perspective to include everybody. We're *all* developing, and we all enter and leave developmental stages — all the way through adulthood — that are characterized by time of life. For you, in the middle of your forties, the developmental phase is not infancy, not childhood or adolescence, not early adulthood or adulthood, but perimenopause. You're in your forties, Gloria, and the forties bring with them certain changes that have an effect on your life. The results of these changes can be delicious satisfaction or maddening discomfort. They can be surprisingly enjoyable or greatly challenging to your sense of well-being. The insomnia, for instance. It seems to be making you miserable in just about all areas of your life."

"You've got it," mumbled Gloria, staring at her knees.

"But see, there's an explanation for it related to your time of life. And furthermore, because we can include that explanation in the possible causes of your insomnia, we can hone in more accurately on an appropriate treatment."

Gloria walked out of my office with confidence that the problem that had been growing over the course of a year was, with a little experimentation, going to be solved. And I was left with a new way of looking at perimenopause. That the very term has only come into use recently is proof in itself that seeing our lives as a continuous process of growth and change has only just begun to take hold. Perimenopause is the frame around a picture that, unframed, was amorphous and hard to understand. Framed in this way, highlighting their unique place in the whole curve of human development, our forties become comprehensible in a whole new way, and our view of ourselves suddenly jumps into much sharper focus.

CHAPTER TWO

Where Are You in the Process?

When a woman comes in to see me with concerns about whether she is "menopausal," the first thing I review with her is the difference between menopause and perimenopause. Many women are confused about this, and why wouldn't they be? We certainly didn't grow up hearing the word *perimenopause,* much less knowing what it means.

This chapter will take you through a careful review of changes in your body's important functions. If you compare your checklist of symptoms, changes, and experiences with your best friend's, keep in mind that yours may be very different, even though you both may be perimenopausal. These variations are part of what confuses us. We have been led to believe that we must have a certain set of symptoms and specific criteria in order to be officially recognized as belonging to a particular category. In perimenopause, however, there is no one box into which all of us neatly fit.

The exercises we'll go through in this chapter are valuable for several important reasons. First, it's worthwhile for you to *take time* to become more familiar with your body as it changes. Reviewing your history and thinking about where you are today will give you an organized picture of what you know and will help you identify the questions you need to have answered. Second, these exercises will help you readjust your thinking about how your body functions and changes, reminding you that there is no "formula" or "prescription" for perimenopause that will describe all women. Third, the retrospective questions are very helpful in pinpointing when the changes you are experiencing began. (Women are often very surprised to realize that their subtle changes started long before they came to see me for help.) But perhaps most important, spending time reflecting on what is different for you now physically and emotionally will renew and strengthen your trust in yourself. It's empowering to realize, "Yes, I do know what's going on with my body and my psyche. No, I'm not imagining these symptoms, and I'm not just stressed out."

If you came in to see me in person or had an appointment with me by phone, we would start by exploring the "Your Place in the Perimenopausal Process" questions together. You'll notice that the questions go far beyond those you've answered on dozens of doctors' forms, such as your age at first period, number of pregnancies, and so forth. Of course, that information is an important part of your history, but now I want to give you the opportunity to describe your perimenopausal changes in greater depth and with more nuances.

You need to discover more about the interwoven changes in your body and mind that are unique to you in your forties. That's why it's important to consider "all" of you — not just the cluster of physical symptoms — when you do this exercise. Your emotions about your changes and the ways in which you may be redefining your identity will also come into play as you respond to the questions.

Finally, this exercise will give you a clearer sense of where you are in the perimenopausal process, what changes you've experienced, and which ones may lie ahead. Most important, writing down specific symptoms and changes is a key step toward recognizing the appropriate solutions. So give yourself as much time as you need, and don't be concerned if there are some dates or details you can't remember.

1. Have your menstrual cycles changed?

2. If yes, how? Are they longer? Shorter?

3. Is your flow heavier, lighter, or the same as it has been in the past?

4. Are your periods regular, or have they become more unpredictable recently?

5. When did the changes in your cycle begin? Last month? Several months ago? Last year? Several years ago? (If the time frame seems hazy, it sometimes helps to think about how you felt last summer, or last holiday season, for example, and compare that with how you feel today.)

6. Is sexual intercourse more difficult because of vaginal dryness?

7. Does your sex drive seem to be changing?

8. Do you notice that you are very interested in sex at times and totally uninterested at other times?

9. Does your lack of interest in sex seem unexplainable?

10. Do you feel that your memory is less sharp than it used to be?

11. Have you walked into a room and wondered what you were doing there?

12. Have you forgotten someone's name even if it is someone you know well or see often?

13. Have you found yourself in a meeting, unable to remember what is on the agenda?

14. Do you have less overall stamina than you once had?

15. Do you urinate more frequently?

16. Do you lose urine when you sneeze, cough, or laugh?

17. Is the need to urinate more urgent and sudden?

18. Do you have more frequent bladder infections?

19. Is your skin drier than it used to be?

20. Do your facial wrinkles seem more noticeable?

21. What about your body — is it changing shape?

22. Is it more difficult to stay at your ideal weight?

23. Do you know how old your mother was when she went through "menopause"?

24. If not, what about an older sister or maternal aunt?

25. Are your moods more changeable than you would like?

26. Do you become tearful, irritable, or anxious more often?

27. Have friends, co-workers, or family members noticed or remarked about your moods?

28. Are you waking up at night soaking wet with perspiration?

29. Have you turned beet red in the face during the day from a hot flash?

30. Do you have heart palpitations?

31. Do you find yourself lying wide awake in the middle of the night, only to drift off to sleep about an hour before your alarm is set to go off?

32. Do you have headaches?

33. Are your headaches more frequent or severe than they have been in the past?

34. Do your headaches occur in any pattern, such as before, during, or just after your period?

WHAT'S NEXT?

Now that you've had a chance to review your history and think about what's happening, let me reassure you that many of the changes you have just described are present in most perimenopausal women. While the symptoms may be confusing and surprising, they are a normal part of the process. That's not to say by any means that you have to live with symptoms or feelings that interfere with your life — on the contrary. But this is a time to reverse any adversarial thinking you may have about changing. You can be with yourself in your forties in a way that is companionable, much as you would be with a valued and trusted friend. Yes, you're changing, but you can meet those changes with a fit, resilient body and an outlook that sees a promise of good things to come and that affirms who you are.

The questions you've just answered aren't intended to "diagnose" perimenopause or label its symptoms. Rather, they provide you with a personal inventory of your experiences and a perimenopausal self-portrait. That was the case with Janice, a 45-year-old professional woman who came to my clinic and responded to these same questions. She hadn't explicitly noted any of the changes she experienced, and she was startled by some of the answers she gave. "I never stopped to think about the fact that my cycle actually started changing last Christmas. That means I've been going through some of these changes for over a year already."

Not until Janice sat down with her calendars from the past two years did she realize that not only her periods but her emotions, at times, had been shifting for longer than she thought. Her monogrammed, leather-bound diaries were crowded with appointments reflecting her personal and professional priorities. Interestingly, when she saw a conference on her calendar from last spring, she remembered getting her period while she was on the road and being totally unprepared for it. She remembered her stepson's graduation from high school, but only as she reviewed her calendar with the goal of tracing her own changes did she recall trying to stifle her yawns as "Pomp and Circumstance" played. "I hadn't slept for two or three nights before that—my insomnia was unrelenting," she recalled.

Janice flipped through her calendar for several more months until she came to a Tuesday in October for which her notation read "first budget review." "I've been preparing the annual budget ever since I was promoted to my current position five years ago," she told me. "But last fall I had so much trouble with the numbers—they were swimming on the spreadsheets. I actually got my eyes checked, but the ophthalmologist said the prescription for my glasses was fine." As the picture of her perimenopausal changes started to fall into place, Janice laughed at herself for thinking her eyesight had been to blame for her mental fogginess. "I see now that my sleep has been sporadic, and that I've had trouble concentrating during the day on and off for many months," she said. The budget she submitted was ultimately approved, "but I sweated that one out," Janice said. "Even though this is my area of expertise, I was deeply anxious about my work. I also felt depressed, because I started to question my own competence."

For Janice, hot flashes during the day made "sweating out the budget" more than a figure of speech. "Look how many times I have 'drop off dry cleaning' on my list over the last six months!" she exclaimed. "My office gets afternoon sun and tends to be warm, but now that I think of it, I've been peeling off my jacket many times in the morning lately because I feel like I'm in a furnace."

Like Janice, you may have found that as your life moves on, you don't always have time to tune in to what's going on with your body. Many of us keep such a relentlessly busy pace that it's easy to overlook or deny signs of perimenopause. Even though I have worked in the field of women's health for eighteen years, I overlooked some of my own changes. Like me, you may have wondered whether certain symptoms you had were really happening ("Is this really a hot flash, or is this room just stifling?"), or like Janice, who thought she needed new glasses when she couldn't concentrate on her spreadsheets, you may have searched for an explanation that was actually unrelated to the fact that your body, mind, and spirit are moving through this transition.

Knowing about your symptoms may make experiences that you or others formerly dismissed as vague or inconsequential seem more valid. Certain issues that you were reluctant to acknowledge even to yourself, or to mention to your health care provider, may have also come to light. Remember that your intuition about your body is very sound, and you can trust your wisdom when something seems "different" or "not quite right."

After Janice and I reviewed her symptoms, we agreed that sleep disturbances and hot flashes were the issues she most wanted to address. Then we started looking over her lifestyle to identify steps she could take immediately, starting that day. She wanted to sleep better, feel more alert, and get her hot flashes under control as soon as possible.

As I do with my patients, I want to take a look, with you, at how you live. Continuing to assess your lifestyle issues will help you get ready to make some necessary changes — changes that are not about deprivation or sacrifice but about taking control and feeling more in charge of your life right away. Keeping the bigger picture in focus, let's look at changes that add strength, vitality, and a sense of accomplishment to your life during this transitional time.

EATING PATTERNS

35. Do you eat breakfast?
36. If so, how many times a week, and what foods do you eat?
37. If not, why not?
38. Do you eat lunch?
39. What kinds of foods do you eat for lunch?
40. Do you eat dinner?
41. What kinds of foods do you eat for dinner?
42. Do you have any snacks at midmorning or midafternoon?
43. What kinds of foods do you eat for snacks?

CAFFEINE CONSUMPTION

44. Do you drink caffeinated beverages (coffee, hot or iced tea, caffeinated sodas)?
45. How many times a day do you have a caffeinated drink?
46. What times of day do you drink caffeine?

ALCOHOL INTAKE

47. Do you drink alcohol?
48. How many drinks per week?
49. How much do you drink at a time?
50. What type of alcohol do you drink?
51. Does anyone in your family have a problem with alcohol?

EXERCISE HABITS

52. Do you exercise?

53. What types of exercise do you prefer?

54. How often do you exercise?

55. How long do you exercise?

56. When was the last time you exercised?

NUTRITIONAL SUPPLEMENTS

57. Do you take vitamins?

58. What kind of vitamins do you take?

59. In what amount?

60. How regularly do you take vitamins?

61. Are you taking other nutritional supplements?

62. What kind of supplements?

63. In what amount?

64. How regularly do you take supplements?

STRESS LEVEL

65. Do you work outside the home?

66. How many hours a week do you work?

67. Is your stress primarily from work?

68. Are you in a stressful personal relationship with a significant other?

69. If you have children, do you have stressful concerns with them?

70. Are you having significant financial concerns?

71. Is a significant life change such as a divorce, a death in the family, a move, a new job, or a change in financial status on your mind right now?

PERSONAL/FAMILY HISTORY

72. Is there a history of heart disease in your family?

73. If so, which family member(s) had heart disease?

74. At what age?

75. Has either of your parents had a bone fracture from osteoporosis?

76. At what age?

77. Has your grandmother, mother, sister, or aunt had breast cancer?

78. If so, what was the treatment, and how is that person's health today?

79. Any other concerns about your family's health history?

CHARTING

80. Do you chart your symptoms on a daily calendar?

81. How long have you been charting?

82. Have any patterns emerged that are significant?

83. Have you shared your chart with your health care provider?

ACTION PLANS

If you were sitting with me right now, and I knew the answers to the questions you have just answered, our next step would be to put together an action plan appropriate for your unique needs. To give you a concrete example of how an action plan is put together, we'll continue Janice's story, and then we'll meet two other perimenopausal women. By learning about their lives, getting to know them, and sharing their ups and downs as they progress through perimenopause, you'll see different ways of making informed decisions and controlling physical and emotional symptoms.

JANICE, CONTINUED

Organized and efficient, Janice would spend part of each weekend planning menus for her family for the following week. She walked thirty minutes during her lunch break on Mondays, Wednesdays, and Fridays. She also supplemented her healthy diet with a multivitamin and calcium daily. Her work was a challenge that, for the most part, she enjoyed.

Right now, the primary stresses in Janice's life were her own changing physical and emotional situation, and her mother, who at 73 was showing signs of forgetfulness: "She calls and tells me the same thing several times. I say, 'Yes, Mom, you mentioned that last week when we spoke,' and I can tell she doesn't remember." As the oldest daughter, Janice felt responsible for making sure her mother was evaluated by a physician, but she also worried about how she would help manage her mother's needs from several hundred miles away. During her sleepless nights, her thoughts often turned to her mother. "It's hard for me to face that she's getting older," Janice explained, "because everyone always said she looked and acted twenty years younger than her age. Besides, the fact that she's aging means that I'm in a different place in my life too."

Janice described herself as a "a cautious and methodical person who doesn't rush into anything." The action plan we developed together to suit her personality and lifestyle included taking these steps in a two-week period:

+ Take calcium citrate in the evening instead of the morning (1500 mg). Out of habit, she was taking her calcium and multivitamin every morning after breakfast. Because some women report sleeping more soundly when they take calcium before bed, I recommended that she make this simple change in her routine to see if it would help with her insomnia.

+ Take ginkgo biloba for her mental fogginess. An extract of leaves from this ancient tree species appears to increase cerebral blood flow, producing improved memory and mental performance. (See chapter 7 for more on ginkgo.) With its vascular effects, ginkgo is commonly prescribed in Europe to treat a variety of conditions. In Janice's case, I recommended that she begin by taking 120 mg of ginkgo biloba daily (40 mg three times a day). Most health food stores and some groceries carry it.

+ Have her estrogen, progesterone, and testosterone levels measured using saliva testing. Saliva testing would give us a picture of these baseline hormone levels that might be more precise than blood testing. (See chapter 3 for a more detailed explanation of saliva testing.) I gave Janice the name of a laboratory specializing in saliva hormone testing.

✦ Take a low dose of black cohosh (one 20 mg tablet, twice a day) to manage her hot flashes. Black cohosh is a plant that contains phytoestrogens (*phyto* means "plant"). Widely used in Europe for the last forty years, it has been shown to relieve hot flashes, and there is some evidence that it can relieve depression and vaginal atrophy. It is available by prescription, or over the counter in some health food stores and specialized pharmacies as the product Remifemin. Janice said she felt comfortable trying black cohosh and ginkgo biloba for two weeks to see what effect these plant-based remedies would have on her symptoms.

✦ Check in with her primary care physician. Janice had had a physical eight months before that showed she was in excellent health. But she did not discuss her hot flashes or her difficulty concentrating with her doctor then. "I'm not sure why, because she's someone I respect and she's very easy to talk to," Janice said. "I think I was convinced that if I didn't talk about my difficulty concentrating, it would go away."

I recommended that Janice let her physician know she was having her hormone levels measured with saliva testing, to be sure that the doctor got the results and kept them with Janice's medical records. Janice also wanted to mention to her physician that she was going to try black cohosh. I let Janice know that I would be available to talk with her doctor about any of the perimenopausal issues we had discussed.

✦ Chart her symptoms on her daily calendar. A simple charting method is to track the two physical and two emotional symptoms that are most troublesome, in Janice's case hot flashes, sleeplessness, difficulty concentrating, and anxiety. Each day, I said, she should assign each of these symptoms a number from 0 to 5 that reflected her experience that day. Zero would mean no symptoms, and 5 would mean severe.

DAILY CHART

Psychological Symptoms

     1._____

     2._____

Physical Symptoms

     1._____

     2._____

Ratings: 0 (absence of symptom), 1, 2, 3, 4, 5

     First day _____ (date)

Psychological Symptom #1 _____

                        #2 _____

Physical Symptom   #1 _____

                        #2 _____

Comments: _____

_____

_____

_____

_____

_____

◆ Check back with me in two weeks, so that we could review her chart. Janice's objective record of her symptoms and their response to the herbs, along with the results of her hormone tests, would help us decide if she needed more treatment. If so, we'd explore traditional medications as well as additional complementary or alternative remedies. She might not need any further intervention right away — plenty of women do just fine with self-care. But if she did, I wanted to be sure she knew about all of her choices.

Janice left my office feeling that she had more clarity about what was happening with her body, more understanding of her choices, and more resolve that her symptoms could be dealt with effectively. She also felt empowered and energized about moving forward with her two-week game plan.

Sharon

A married "at-home mom," Sharon was a 48-year-old mother of two preteens and an adopted toddler. She was very involved in her children's school activities and in her community.

Sharon's list of symptoms included depression, bloating, forgetfulness, insomnia, and hot flashes. She still had periods, but they were much closer together than they were three or four years ago. Her flow was lighter, and she was concerned about this change, thinking it might signal that something was wrong.

A very physically active woman, Sharon played tennis two to three times a week and ran at least four times a week. She was in excellent condition, but her diet needed a little evening out. She was accustomed to taking care of her family, and she made sure her children and husband had healthy snacks and meals. But for herself, she did not always eat the nutritious meals she conscientiously prepared for them. "Sometimes I'm standing in the kitchen nervously eating an aging and syrupy piece of toast my toddler abandoned hours ago," she told me. "Or I'll demolish six cookies while I'm making a salad for the family, but then I won't eat dinner. I also tend to rely on coffee to pick me up three or four times a day."

Sharon had been raised on a farm and grew up eating straight from the garden, which was probably why she believed vitamins aren't really necessary if you eat good food. She enjoyed cooking and baking, and she prided herself on her creativity with food.

When her husband recently experienced a life-threatening illness, Sharon felt as if her life were "coming apart." His prognosis was good, but she had residual anxiety from this scary time and felt fatigued after acting as the rock of Gibraltar for the family during his illness.

Sharon was a "can do" type of person, who relied on her own strength to meet any situation in her life. Right now, she wanted to try to handle her anxiety, depression, and hot flashes without taking medication. I recommended that, to begin with, we focus on her diet and on reducing her stress level, taking these initial steps:

- ✦ Add soy to her diet. Soy products, like the plant black cohosh, contain phytoestrogens. (See chapter 7 for more on the role of phytoestrogens in managing perimenopausal symptoms.) Soy is particularly high in the type of phytoestrogens called isoflavones. Studies show that soy lowers cholesterol, increases bone density (in animals), and possibly decreases the risk of breast cancer, although the evidence here is not entirely conclusive.

    The isoflavones in soy foods may also benefit perimenopausal women by alleviating hot flashes and vaginal dryness. Researchers don't yet understand everything about how phytoestrogens work in the body, but one theory suggests that these substances may "bind" to estrogen receptors. The body then reacts as if there really were estrogen in these receptor sites. (Japanese women, whose diet is usually very high in soy foods, complain of far fewer symptoms of perimenopause than women in Western countries.)

- ✦ Work up to 50 mg of isoflavones per day. The amount of isoflavones in different soy products varies, and not all soy products list isoflavone content on their labels. Soy oil and soy sauce contain few isoflavones, while tofu, tempeh, and roasted soy nuts are high in isoflavones. One and a third cups of soy milk or a little over half a cup of either tempeh, tofu, or roasted soy nuts per day will provide approximately 50 mg of isoflavones. Sharon was also interested in experimenting with using soy flour as an ingredient in the pancakes and muffins she often made. I suggested she take a look at *Earl Mindell's Soy Miracle*, which contains a good section on cooking with soy.

✦ Eat more frequently throughout the day, preferably every two to three hours. Since she had a toddler at home, I suggested that when she was feeding her a snack, she too eat half a banana with a handful of whole-wheat crackers, or a piece of low-fat cheese with half a pear.

✦ Supplement her diet with a good multivitamin as well as a B-complex vitamin containing at least 100 mg of B$_6$. Vitamin B$_6$ is a natural diuretic that can help reduce bloating. The B family of vitamins acts on the central nervous system, which is why they are sometimes called "stress tabs." ProCycle or ProCycle Gold with calcium are options for perimenopausal women, since these vitamin, mineral, and trace-element supplements have a strong B-complex component.

✦ Cut her caffeine consumption in half every four days. Since she was having three or four cups of coffee a day now, four days from now Sharon would cut down to one and a half or two cups, until she could drink less than a cup a day without getting a caffeine withdrawal headache. I let her know that if she did develop a headache even as she cut down slowly, taking two or three swallows of coffee would usually alleviate this symptom. I recommended that she drink her coffee before noon.

Keeping caffeine consumption at a reasonable level is a fairly standard health recommendation by now, but this advice has even more weight for perimenopausal women. Excess caffeine can worsen hormonally related insomnia, and its dilating effects can contribute to hot flashes.

✦ Consider another means of stress reduction, such as yoga and stretching, in addition to her regular forms of exercise. Sharon relied on exercise to reduce her anxiety, and her runs and tennis games were a very important part of her life. But when she felt anxious or pressured, she sometimes ran for longer and longer distances, which might contribute to her fatigue. She acknowledged that she might literally be trying to "run away" from the pressures of home and her husband's recent illness. I gave her a book on yoga, and she said she was willing to look through it and experiment with two or three of the exercises at least twice before our next meeting.

+ Have her estrogen, progesterone, and testosterone levels measured with saliva testing.

+ Begin charting her symptoms.

+ Return for a follow-up visit in two weeks.

When Sharon had first come into my office, she looked a bit teary, but she left with a much brighter expression on her face. The tools we identified were appropriate for her—her enjoyment of cooking fit well with the plan to add foods with phytoestrogens to her meals. She was excited and encouraged to think that we could actually get a "hormonal picture" of her situation with the saliva tests. And while balancing running with slower, more meditative yoga movements seemed novel to her, she was nevertheless intrigued with the idea of spending quiet time with herself.

Mary

Mary was 42 and unmarried but in a serious relationship. She was a high-powered professional in a field that had only recently opened up to include more than a few women. She still had a regular menstrual cycle with a period every twenty-seven days, but she skipped a period two months ago. Some "new" problems had emerged for Mary: irritability, anxiety, sleeplessness, weight gain, decreased sex drive, and vaginal dryness. "This couldn't be 'the change,' could it?" she asked me in amazement.

Mary's recent routine physical had included a blood test for follicle-stimulating hormone, which showed a normal level (under 20 ng/ml). I explained that FSH levels are only part of the picture, and that women in their forties often have FSH levels that vary from month to month. (Doctors sometimes use FSH measurement as an indicator of whether a woman is menopausal; see chapter 3.)

Mary's typical day at the office started at seven A.M. and proceeded through a solid schedule of appointments, meetings, and phone calls. She rarely left before seven P.M. and spent many Saturdays working. "I get my work ethic from my dad," she said. "He worked very hard all his life — maybe too hard. He died unexpectedly of a heart attack when he was fifty-five, before he had a chance to retire and enjoy himself." Mary admitted that the stress of her job had been getting to her lately: "The everyday pressures seem harder to handle even though what I do hasn't changed."

Sometimes Mary started her day with a doughnut and coffee from the corner store in her neighborhood, and she ate a lot of rich food at lunches with her clients. She usually didn't eat dinner until after eight P.M., and frequently that meal consisted of leftover pizza. She did take a vitamin supplement and had been taking calcium citrate (the type of calcium most easily absorbed by our bodies) since she was in her midthirties. Exercise wasn't part of her life. She said the demands of her career didn't leave her enough time.

Mary and I agreed that changing her eating and exercise habits would be challenging and might take some time. In the meantime she seemed almost desperate. "I'm so anxious and irritable," she told me. "I spend too much energy during the day trying to calm myself down, trying not to bite someone's head off, or apologizing because I've already said something abrasive."

Mary and I talked about the fact that she might be a candidate for hormone replacement therapy (HRT) for three key reasons. First, she wanted to feel better right away, and some women do find that symptoms of sleeplessness, anxiety, and irritability are alleviated quickly when they supplement their body's supply of hormones (estrogen, progesterone, and testosterone). Second, she had a family history of heart disease, and HRT provides cardiac protection. Third, it was unlikely that Mary would "relearn" her eating habits or take on an exercise routine overnight.

As a first step, taking natural progesterone might break the cycle of symptoms that were making Mary feel desperate and harried. Depending on the outcome of her hormone tests, we would evaluate whether estriol, a type of estrogen that targets the female genitourinary tract, would be appropriate for the vaginal dryness that was bothering her. (Estriol is sometimes called the "weak" or "forgotten" estrogen — it does not stimulate breast or uterine tissue and is often overlooked as a treatment option for vaginal dryness and stress incontinence.) We'd also consider balancing Mary's hormones and putting the spark back in her dwindling libido by supplementing her with a low dose of natural testosterone.

Trying hormone supplementation to bring her symptoms under control was just one of Mary's overall health goals. Over time, as she regained control of her body and emotions, we would work on developing healthier lifestyle habits for her. Right now, the strategy that best suited her hectic life included these action steps:

+ Have her estrogen, progesterone, testosterone, and cortisol levels measured in saliva within two days, before any medical intervention began. In addition to determining whether Mary might be experiencing any reproductive hormone fluctuations, we wanted to see if the hormone cortisol was elevated, which can happen when a person is under duress. Prolonged elevation of cortisol levels can lead to a suppression of certain immune functions.

+ Take a fifteen-minute walk at least twice on separate days during the following two weeks. To make time for these walks, Mary would limit herself to returning only ten phone calls and would give the other calls to her assistant to return. That way she could buy herself the essential half an hour. She would take her walking shoes to work so that she could easily head out for a walk.

+ Begin charting her symptoms.

+ Note what she was eating on her symptom chart, so she could see for herself what kinds of food she was eating and when.

+ Meet with me again in two weeks. Mary made a commitment to herself not to cancel our follow-up appointment and reschedule for a later date.

For my part, I decided to take several steps to help Mary:

+ Contact Mary's health care provider about starting her on 200 mg a day of natural progesterone during this menstrual cycle. (Mary was on day 5 of a twenty-seven-day cycle; progesterone can start on day 13.) Natural progesterone, which is derived from yams and soybeans, frequently relieves symptoms of irritability, anxiety, and sleeplessness during the first cycle in which it is used.

+ Since Mary's weight concerned her, ask her health care provider if her thyroid level had been measured recently. If not, we might want to order this test to determine if a thyroid imbalance could be affecting her weight.

+ Set a date to review the results of Mary's hormone tests with her health care provider, so we could discuss whether adding estrogen and testosterone to her regimen would be beneficial.

Mary went home feeling more hopeful that *she* was in charge of her body, instead of the reverse. The hands-on suggestions gave her confidence that she could put an end to her feeling that her life was out of kilter. She could start feeling that she was in control again.

We'll follow Janice, Sharon, and Mary's stories throughout this book to see what worked for them, what didn't, and how their situations changed. I assured each of them that they could call me before our next appointment if they had questions or concerns.

I hope you will allow yourself to use this book as if you and I were working together, just as I was with Janice, Sharon, and Mary, because that is in fact what we are doing. We've started with the basics here, just as we would if we were sitting down face to face. I encourage you to chart your symptoms for the next two weeks, noting the ones that are interfering most with your life, and using the sample format on page 23 or a variation that is comfortable for you.

We'll move on to address more complex and technical concerns, but if you have an urgent question that you need help with immediately, you can call my toll-free number (1-800-418-4040), e-mail me at womenshealth@hotmail.com with your personal questions, or check in with my website (http://www.menopause-pms.com) to get more information.

Perimenopausal symptoms often fluctuate—you may develop new symptoms or find that the ones you have now get better, seemingly on their own. Often these variations come with no warning, for no rhyme or reason, and their uneven cadence can be disconcerting. So don't be surprised, dismayed, or confused if what you write or describe today is very different at some point in the future. As your body goes through this natural transition, it can take time to establish a rhythm that seems stable. Be assured that there is no "right" or "predictable" way to go through perimenopause. Our goal is to move through this transition with good health, a sense of humor, and abiding dignity and empowerment.

CHAPTER THREE

The Hormonal Landscape

*W*hen we travel by car or train on a literal journey, we sometimes need to stop and look at a map or ask for directions, depending on our style. This chapter will help you get your bearings on your path through the hormonal landscape — where *you're* in charge of navigating, where the map is unique to you, and where you decide which steps are best for you. In particular, I'll describe how the hormonal landscape changes during the transitional decade of our forties. We'll see where Janice, Sharon, and Mary were on their own perimenopausal journey. You may recognize similarities with your situation, and you'll learn more about identifying and managing your own changes.

A basic understanding of how our hormones work is necessary to be able to interpret the changes we experience, explain them to our families, and evaluate our choices thoroughly and carefully. After all, the more you know about how your body matures, the more secure you'll feel that nothing is going "wrong" with you, and the better equipped you'll be to form an effective support system with your family, friends, and health care providers.

Of course, to explain all of the complex interactions our hormones have with each other and with other chemicals produced in our bodies and brains, I would have to write a weighty medical textbook. Instead, my purpose here is to give you a basic overview of the subtle and elegant ways our bodies produce and use hormones. "Just the basics" will help you understand how our bodies work hormonally and allow you to be your own best friend as your hormonal functions change.

Hormones are chemicals that are produced by our endocrine glands (like ovaries). They have an intimate relationship with chemicals produced by our brains, called neurotransmitters, such as serotonin, dopamine, and norepinephrine. We've all heard the negative expression "raging hormones," but let's not lose sight of the fact that our female hormones enhance our physical and mental well-being, help our bodies perform all kinds of elaborate functions, and nourish not only our reproductive organs but our skin, hair, bones, heart, and brain! As women's health expert Michelle Harrison, M.D., says, "Our hormones don't make us sick. Our hormones keep us well."

Our bodies are very sensitive to hormonal effects, and if our hormones are out of balance, the hormonal wellness that Dr. Harrison talks about can be threatened. We may feel as if we're roller-coasting up and down steep cliffs, or trying to keep our footing on some very rocky ground while wearing three-inch heels.

As we view the hormonal landscape in this chapter, we'll pay special attention to four key hormones: estrogen and progesterone, which are produced by the ovaries; and follicle-stimulating hormone (FSH) and luteinizing hormone (LH), both produced by the brain. (We'll talk about testosterone and other hormones in a later chapter.)

We tend to think of the path through our hormonal landscape as beginning at menarche (when we had our first period). The first information many of us received about our hormones may have been in that discreet little booklet about menstruation handed out in grade school. It may surprise you, but in fact our journey through the hormonal landscape starts at birth.

Female infants are born with approximately two million potential eggs (follicles) in our ovaries. By the time we reach puberty, usually at age 12 or 13, we have only 400,000 follicles left. No one understands where these follicles go or exactly why eighty percent of them vanish, but they do.

As adult women, we fully understand the value of preparation and planning ahead—organizing dozens of things on a daily basis for our families, jobs, and other commitments. The same advance planning occurs in nature as our bodies prepare to reach our biological milestones. Our hormonal changes over time are neither sudden nor precipitous but gradual.

Like menopause, menarche—the onset of our first period—is not a sudden hormonal event but one outcome of a very deliberate process. Our ovaries were already producing estrogen during our prepubescent years, at ages 9, 10, and 11, to get our bodies ready for the reproductive years ahead.

Sharon, the at-home mother we met earlier, was startled when her daughter, a third grader, started to develop breasts. "She's only nine years old. I can't believe it! The other day we ended up sharing the bathroom as she was finishing her shower. I noticed the beginning of breasts, and it really took me by surprise. Does this mean she'll start menstruating soon?" Sharon asked me.

Sharon's young daughter's body was definitely showing signs of early hormonal stimulation. But it didn't necessarily mean that she would start her period any day. Sharon herself had experienced menarche at age 10. Chances are her daughter would follow that pattern fairly closely. In fact, most women's reproductive history (the timing and pattern of menarche, perimenopause, and menopause) is very similar to their mothers'. Sharon and I also talked about how this would be a wonderful time for her to discuss menstruation with her daughter.

At 48, Sharon's own body was changing along with her daughter's, at a different point on the same female developmental arc. As her body gradually wound down its reproductive function, her once-predictable menstrual cycle had become irregular. In fact, her daughter's changes tuned her in more closely to her own changed relationship with herself as a perimenopausal woman.

"There's a bittersweet feeling about seeing my daughter start to mature at the same time I'm observing my own body changes," Sharon said. "The timing seems appropriate, though. It makes sense that I'm about to pass the torch to her, even though I find myself deep in thought as I watch her growing up."

THE MENSTRUAL CYCLE DURING PERIMENOPAUSE

As part of "passing the torch," Sharon would help her young daughter understand her body's gentle metamorphosis into womanhood and, in the process, teach her about menstruation. Regardless of whether you will be explaining menstruation to a young girl in your forties, it makes sense to review the menstrual cycle, since your own changing hormonal patterns can alter your cycle and directly affect the way you look, feel, and think.

The hormonal landscape begins to look different in perimenopause. The once-predictable rise in estrogen to dominance during the first half of each menstrual cycle is not as stable as it once was. Progesterone, the dominant hormone during the second half of the cycle, may also be out of balance. We may get a period totally unexpectedly, as Janice did when she was out of town attending a conference. Or we may skip periods, as Mary did for two months. Some women, like Sharon, have more subtle interruptions in their menstrual cycle, such as a lighter flow or periods that come more frequently than every twenty-eight days. Sharon also experienced depression, hot flashes, and fatigue. These hormonal changes can leave us feeling out of control, especially if mood swings, depression, or other symptoms hit us at times of the month when we don't expect them.

In fact, many women I work with who are in their forties miss the predictability of the menstrual cycle when it begins to change. Predictability is an important piece of our lives, and when it diminishes, its absence can be very unsettling.

In the past, you may have counted on being at your best during the first half of your cycle—you may have felt that sense of energy, well-being, and revitalization that some women say they feel when their period ends. Or you may have learned to expect (and cope with) premenstrual irritability, food cravings, or other symptoms because you knew they would end when your period started. But when perimenopausal hormone shifts cause symptoms to show up seemingly at random, you may feel betrayed by your body's infidelity to its previous rhythm.

Let's briefly revisit what is involved in the menstrual cycle—which hormones do what and when. First, it's called a cycle because it really doesn't end—it just keeps going around and around like a clock. At various times during the cycle, different hormones are doing their job.

Day 1, the first day of the menstrual flow, starts the first of two phases of the menstrual cycle. The body has just begun to slough off the lining of the uterus (the endometrium) because a pregnancy did not occur. This first phase, called the follicular phase, lasts from day 1 to approximately day 14, just before ovulation occurs.

In the follicular phase, the estrogen level starts to rise, while the progesterone level remains low. During this phase the brain signals the body to produce follicle-stimulating hormone. FSH encourages a follicle (one of the 400,000 immature eggs stored in the ovaries) to mature or ripen. The actual release of the ripened follicle from the ovary is the process called ovulation.

The hormone responsible for triggering the release of the ripened egg or follicle is called luteinizing hormone (LH). Some women can tell when they are ovulating because they feel a sensation on their right or left side, depending on which ovary is releasing an egg that month. This sensation, called Mittelschmerz, is often described as a cramping or pinching feeling, and it can last anywhere from a few moments to a few hours. Some women also report an increase in vaginal discharge when they ovulate.

Take a moment to think about whether you have noticed your own ovulation at any point in your life. Ovulation, which usually happens sometime between ten and fourteen days into the menstrual cycle, may become erratic during perimenopause. This is one reason women in their forties have a high rate of unplanned pregnancies, second only to teenagers. (Unless you have not had a period for twelve consecutive months, you need to continue to use birth control if you do not want to become pregnant.) On the other hand, some women in their forties who are trying to conceive have difficulty—they may be ovulating irregularly,

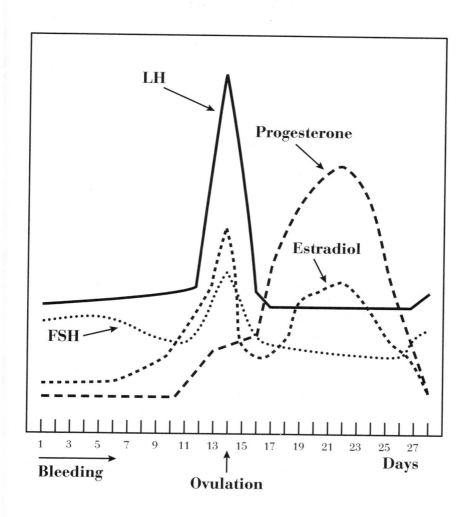

Hormone levels during the cycle

SOURCE: BONNICK, S.L. *THE OSTEOPOROSIS HANDBOOK.* DALLAS: TAYLOR PUBLISHING, 1997.

at times of the month when they don't expect it, or not at all some months. With the release of the ripened follicle, the second half of the menstrual cycle, or luteal phase, begins.

LOW ESTROGEN = DIFFERENT SYMPTOMS

As we enter the perimenopausal phase of our lives, our levels of estrogen and other hormones begin to fluctuate. These hormonal shifts play out very differently in individual women.

You'll recall that Janice, Sharon, and Mary all had their levels of estrogen and other hormones measured by saliva testing. Although their symptoms and their life situations were very different, their test results all showed certain trends in common, one of which was low estradiol levels.

While we might think of estrogen as just one chemical, estrogen is actually a *category* of hormones. In fact, our bodies make many types of estrogen, three of which are predominant:

1. Estradiol. This potent form of estrogen is produced by the ovaries in larger amounts in fully fertile women. (Women are "fully fertile" once the rhythm of their menstrual cycle is in place and they are ovulating. Young girls usually menstruate *without* ovulating for six months to a year after their first period. The "fully fertile" or reproductive years usually span thirty to thirty-five years of a woman's life.) As women begin perimenopause, their ovaries produce less estradiol. That's what the test results indicate for Janice, Sharon, and Mary. But estradiol is only one part of our hormonal landscape — many other factors also play a part in determining our perimenopausal experiences.

2. Estrone. This type of estrogen, also potent, is produced from the conversion of estradiol. During perimenopause, when the ovaries produce less and less estradiol, a transition is made in which the fat cells start synthesizing estrone. Women who have more fat cells seem to have fewer perimenopausal symptoms. Obviously, this isn't nature's way of saying it's a good idea to be overweight,

but it may be a cautionary note about the health risks of being ultrathin.

3. Estriol. Sometimes called the "forgotten" estrogen, estriol is the weakest of the three major types of estrogen. It is produced from the conversion of estrone and is also produced in very high amounts by the placenta during pregnancy.

PROGESTERONE AND PERIMENOPAUSE

Estrogen has unique properties that enhance our brains and bodies, but our reproductive functioning and overall health lean heavily on the delicate interplay between estrogen and progesterone. Progesterone, which is produced by the ovaries, takes over during the luteal phase (second half of the cycle), while estrogen takes a back seat, its mission accomplished for now. Literally, *progesterone* means "for pregnancy." This hormone causes the uterine lining to become rich and spongy, so a fertilized egg can implant and sustain a pregnancy, if conception has occurred.

Throughout the second half of the menstrual cycle, rising progesterone levels keep the uterine lining intact. When no pregnancy has been achieved, it is progesterone that causes the uterine lining to be sloughed off as menstrual flow. Progesterone drops significantly at the very end of the menstrual cycle (just before a period begins), causing the endometrium to be shed. Without progesterone, we couldn't get pregnant or carry a baby to term. As we age beyond our childbearing years, our bodies respond by producing less progesterone.

When progesterone production diminishes in perimenopause, some women skip periods, then may have periods with an unusually heavy flow. The reduced amount of progesterone in the body no longer triggers the start of the menstrual flow in a predictable, monthly pattern, which is why perimenopausal women often have irregular periods. Lower progesterone levels also explain why the endometrium may build up too much before it sloughs: lack of progesterone means a longer period of time before the uterine lining is shed. Remember Mary, who skipped a period for two months? I would suspect that her progesterone levels were low.

While both estrogen and progesterone decline during peri-menopause, scientists don't know which one begins to drop off first, or if the sequence of their changes is significant. Women in their forties often develop new or intensified PMS-like symptoms (believed to be associated with fluctuations in progesterone) for months or sometimes years before they experience hot flashes (which correlate with a decline in estrogen). This fact suggests that progesterone production slows down first during the perimenopausal transition, although the consequences of declining estrogen certainly get more press.

If future research determines that progesterone in fact does begin to decline *before* estrogen levels fall, several very interesting areas of study will open up: Would supplementing with progesterone early in perimenopause relieve or avoid certain symptoms entirely? Could main-taining the progesterone/estrogen balance possibly delay or eliminate the need for estrogen replacement in some women? We don't have these answers yet, but I believe the questions we raise and the experiences we share will have a profound influence on future scientific investigations.

PROGESTERONE AND MOOD

Progesterone also seems to have a significant bearing on our moods, pro-ducing a calming effect. During pregnancy, progesterone levels soar, reaching levels thirty to fifty times greater than in nonpregnant women. That may be why some women say they feel "very serene" during preg-nancy, or that they have "never felt better."

Lynn's comments on her experience during pregnancy may reflect some of progesterone's effects: "I couldn't believe anyone would ever complain about being pregnant. After the first trimester was over, I felt wonderful. My skin and nails looked so healthy, and my attitude about life was great. As far as I was concerned, everything was right with the world."

Eleven years later, when perimenopausal symptoms of nervous-ness and irritability started to cast shadows on her normally cheerful out-look, she wished she could have "just one day" of the well-being she felt during her last pregnancy. "I toyed with the idea of having another baby for a lot of reasons, not the least of which was wishing I could feel that good again," she told me. Lynn's husband, less nostalgic about the glow of pregnancy and reluctant to readjust his life to care for a newborn again, reacted to her suggestion with shock that was only partially feigned. "His response was 'Not with me, thank you very much,'" Lynn said.

I assured Lynn that pregnancy wasn't her only option for recapturing the well-being she was missing at 43. "Some women find that supplementing with natural micronized progesterone really eases premenstrual anxiety," I told her.

When progesterone levels go out of balance during the second half of the menstrual cycle, some women feel their spirits drop premenstrually. This weepy feeling may result from the fact that progesterone levels haven't risen sufficiently or drop off abruptly during the luteal phase. Another time when progesterone levels fall dramatically is within hours after a woman gives birth. This abrupt hormonal change produces only mild symptoms of depression in some women, while other women feel more acutely depressed after childbirth. In extremely rare cases, women develop postpartum psychosis.

I have found that micronized natural progesterone can be very effective in treating postpartum depression, as well as premenstrual or perimenopausal anxiety. (*Micronized* means "broken down into very tiny particles.") There may be a connection between heightened anxiety or even panic attacks and low levels of progesterone. Mary, who had to will herself to "calm down" during the day, may have been feeling the effects of low progesterone.

In the brain, progesterone binds to certain sites where the "anti-anxiety" brain chemical, GABA, is produced. Progesterone's effect on the brain is similar to the effect of anti-anxiety medications such as Xanax or Valium, which bind to the same sites. In my clinical and personal experience, I have found that progesterone can be a very effective, noninvasive option for managing symptoms of anxiety. This natural and benign medication (micronized natural progesterone is derived from an extract of yams and soybeans) represents an alternative to other potentially addictive anti-anxiety drugs.

Some researchers theorize that insufficient progesterone levels contribute to premenstrual mood changes. Women with premenstrual syndrome (PMS) often report that their moods vary remarkably from the follicular phase (first half) to the luteal phase (second half) of the cycle. This mood change is described by some women as sudden, "as if someone threw a switch in my body." It may be that premenstrual anxiety, irritability, anger, tearfulness, or depression result when a woman's progesterone level falls short of the normal range, is out of balance with estrogen, or both. In perimenopause it is common for women either to experience PMS-like symptoms for the first time or, if they have had these symptoms before, to find that they become noticeably more intense.

This intensification fits the description Mary gave of her symptoms the first time we met: she was so anxious that she had to make a conscious effort to "calm herself down," and she was irritable enough to have to apologize for speaking sharply to her colleagues. The level of her progesterone turned out to be less than 0.05 ng/ml when measured in saliva. (Normal progesterone ranges in saliva are 0.05 to 0.5 ng/ml in women who are still menstruating.) Her physician agreed that it made sense to begin treatment with 200 mg per day of natural micronized progesterone during the luteal phase of her cycle, to see if it would bring her immediate relief. Progesterone supplementation might also regulate the timing of her menstrual cycle.

Mary checked in with me two weeks after our first visit — she had started taking micronized natural progesterone the week before, on day 13 of her cycle. "I'm definitely calmer and less irritable — there's a big difference in how I feel," she said.

"Any change in your sex drive?" I asked.

"Well, not really. And I still have the vaginal dryness."

I wasn't surprised to hear that Mary's mood had lifted even after taking natural micronized progesterone for only a week — generally symptoms improve within a few days. I also wasn't surprised to learn that she still felt indifferent about sex and that vaginal dryness persisted —

those symptoms corresponded with the fact that her estradiol (and testosterone) levels were low.

I recommended adding estriol, the "weak" estrogen, to her regimen, beginning with a dose of 0.5 mg vaginal suppositories, twice a week. (Estriol suppositories must be compounded by a pharmacist — they are not made in mass quantities. Prescriptions for this medication are individualized for each woman taking it.) Vaginal tissue that becomes thin and dry due to declining estrogen can take a long time to respond to any form of treatment, which is why I thought it was important to address this symptom right away. I said I would talk with Mary's doctor about this option.

Janice, too, also had low progesterone levels, although not as low as Mary's. Low estradiol might account for Janice's sleeplessness and difficulty concentrating, but low progesterone might contribute to the disproportionate anxiety she felt about submitting the annual budget, a task she had performed many times before with ease. I would watch her progress as she took black cohosh root (Remifemin) and ginkgo biloba to alleviate the hot flashes and mental fuzziness that were troubling her most.

In Sharon's case, her progesterone test in saliva showed she too had an insufficient level of this hormone. For now, she preferred to continue with her lifestyle approach to managing her perimenopausal symptoms: adding soy to her diet and learning more about yoga as a stress-reduction measure. "Just knowing what was going on with my hormones made a huge difference for me," Sharon said.

HORMONE TESTING: OLD AND NEW

How important is it to know exactly how much estrogen, progesterone, FSH, and other hormones are circulating in our body at one time? What will these measurements tell us? There isn't one simple answer to these questions. In fact, expert opinion is often polarized between two extremes. Some advocate doing every laboratory test available to see what is going on hormonally, because then at least you have *some* information. Others insist that testing hormones is a waste of time and money because our hormone levels fluctuate too much to give a precise reading. (That was also the primary reason for excluding women from medical research in the past.)

The truth about hormone testing lies somewhere in between. As our bodies start to go through perimenopausal changes, our hormonal levels vary and become less rhythmic. Along with charting physical and emotional symptoms of perimenopause on paper, as Janice, Sharon and Mary were doing, hormone testing is also sometimes used to sharpen the picture of perimenopausal changes.

In the past, physicians often relied on blood tests for estradiol and follicle-stimulating hormone to determine if a woman was "menopausal"—no one talked much about the time *leading up to* menopause until recently. Usually done during the follicular phase, the results of an FSH test indicate a woman's estrogen level. That's because as the body's supply of estrogen goes down, it begins to produce more FSH. It's as if the body were urgently trying to stimulate as many follicles as possible before our reproductive capability ends. Therefore, when the FSH reading is high (over 40), it suggests that estrogen levels are low. Surges in FSH may also produce hot flashes—this hormone is believed to dilate hundreds of tiny capillaries below the skin, causing them to fill with blood suddenly and make us feel uncomfortably overheated or flushed.

However, FSH test results are not always definitive. In Mary's case, her FSH blood test showed a reading below 20, which would indicate that she was *not* perimenopausal but in fact fully fertile. Yet her symptoms were significantly interfering with her personal and professional life, suggesting that something else was going on.

When I talked with Mary's doctor about testing her estrogen, progesterone, testosterone, and cortisol levels in saliva, he was skeptical at first about the value of this additional information but was willing to review the results with me. When he saw that her estrogen, progesterone, and testosterone levels were below normal, he didn't come out and say so directly, but I got the impression that he hadn't expected these results. Given that her FSH level had appeared to be normal only a month or two earlier, he might have expected that her estrogen level in particular would be very different: less than 15 ng/ml, within expected range.

Another patient of mine, Madeleine, who is the same age as Mary, had her FSH level measured because she desperately wanted to get pregnant. Her cycle was becoming unpredictable, and she worried that at 42, time was running out for her.

She had her FSH measured for three consecutive months, and each time the result was very different. The first month her FSH showed her to be in the 20 range, which is considered perimenopausal. A month later, it was low enough to suggest she was fully fertile. The third month—still another result—her FSH was over 40, which suggested that she was menopausal. Is it confusing? Yes, absolutely.

What does it all mean? In Mary's case, one "normal" FSH reading didn't tell the whole story, because other hormones, when measured in saliva, were out of normal ranges. For Madeleine, the variability of her FSH test results actually gave her hope that she could still conceive, signifying that her body might not yet be completely past the reproductive phase, and she persevered in her effort to get pregnant. It took her nine more months, but she did conceive and joyfully gave birth to a healthy baby boy.

NEW HORMONE TEST OPTIONS

While FSH can be measured only in blood, the technology to measure estrogen, progesterone, testosterone, and other hormones using saliva samples is now being applied in very innovative ways. First, let me explain how saliva testing differs from blood testing of hormones.

Saliva testing gives a reading of only the unbound or "free" form of the hormone molecules. This is important because only the free hormone molecules can actually act on cells in the body. The free hormone level is probably only two to five percent of the total amount of the hormone in the body, according to experts at Aeron LifeCycles, a California laboratory specializing in saliva testing.

Blood testing, on the other hand, measures both the free and the "bound" hormone molecules, and it doesn't always distinguish between the two. As the name implies, bound hormone molecules remain bound and cannot act on cells. So the blood-test level of a particular hormone doesn't tell us how much of that hormone is available to affect processes in the body. This means that a woman whose blood test shows her to have a normal hormone level could actually have either more or less than the amount of free hormone that her body needs. (For normal ranges in both types of testing, see the "Measuring Hormones in Women" chart.)

MEASURING HORMONES IN WOMEN
Saliva and Blood Levels

HORMONE	NORMAL RANGES IN SALIVA	NORMAL RANGES IN BLOOD
FSH	N/A (FSH IS MEASURED IN SERUM ONLY)	2.5–10.2 mIU/mL (FOLLICULAR) 3.4–63.4 mIU/mL (MIDCYCLE) 1.5–9.1 mIU/mL (LUTEAL)
ESTRADIOL	0.5–5.0 PG/ML (PREMENOPAUSAL) 0.5–1.5 PG/ML	23–145 PG/ML (FOLLICULAR) 112–443 PG/ML (MIDCYCLE) 48–241 PG/ML (LUTEAL)
ESTRIOL	<15 PG/ML	<15 PG/ML
PROGESTERONE	0.05–0.5 NG/ML (PREMENOPAUSAL) <0.05 NG/ML (POSTMENOPAUSAL)	0.1–1.4 NG/ML (FOLLICULAR) 3.3–25.6 NG/ML (LUTEAL)
TESTOSTERONE	20–50 PG/ML (A.M.) 10–20 PG/ML (P.M.)	0.1–0.8 NG/ML
CORTISOL	1.0–10.0 NG/ML (A.M.) 0.5–3.0 NG/ML (P.M.)	4.3–22.4 MCG/DL (A.M.) 3.1–16.7 MCG/DL (P.M.)

SOURCE: AERON LIFECYCLES, MADISON PHARMACY ASSOCIATES.

Saliva testing appears to be much more accurate in measuring estrogen, progesterone, testosterone, and other hormones. These tests are starting to be used by some physicians to adjust hormone replacement dosages. In some cases women and physicians use information from saliva testing to make decisions about other forms of treatment for perimenopausal symptoms. With Janice, Sharon, and Mary, saliva testing resulted in two very important outcomes. First, the results brought them some peace of mind by confirming that their symptoms were not "all in their heads." Second, the objective measure gave them and their health care providers a solid indication of which areas most need attention.

The implications of saliva testing are very, very exciting. To begin with, it is allowing researchers to measure significant patient-to-patient variations not only in baseline hormone levels but in the way hormone supplements are absorbed and metabolized in different dosage forms (oral estrogen versus estrogen in cream form, for example). The work being done by Aeron LifeCycles and Madison Pharmacy Associates shows not only that the *form* of hormone supplement that a woman takes can make a difference but that, in the case of hormone creams or patches, *where* they are applied on the body also affects her hormone levels. For instance, applying very small amounts of progesterone cream to the hands produces significant changes in progesterone levels (as measured in saliva), as opposed to applying it elsewhere on the body, such as on the breasts, abdomen, or inner thighs.

The more precise measurement of hormones through saliva testing could potentially lead to radical reductions in dosages of hormone replacement therapy—to dosages that are *50 to 75 percent lower than current standards*. Mary's situation is one case in point. She was taking 200 mg of natural micronized progesterone a day during the luteal phase of her cycle, but when her physician saw, from saliva testing, that her estradiol levels were less than 0.5 pg/ml, he agreed that supplementing her with a type of estrogen as well might relieve her symptoms of sleeplessness, waning sex drive, and vaginal dryness.

Mary's doctor told me that he normally starts his patients out with 1 mg of Estrace or 0.625 mg of Premarin (both are types of estrogen) and a type of progesterone. But he listened carefully as I talked about estriol, the "weak" or "forgotten" estrogen that can often be used in small amounts (0.5 mg vaginal suppositories, two to three times a week) as a first line of intervention for perimenopausal symptoms of estrogen deficiency.

I faxed him an article about estriol from the *Journal of the American Medical Association*, and he called me back at the end of that day. We discussed adding estriol vaginal suppositories to the 200 mg of micronized natural progesterone Mary was taking daily. (She would take 0.5 mg of estriol in vaginal-suppository form two days a week all month long, but progesterone only from day 13 of her cycle until she got her period.)

He expressed concern about the fact that this low dose of estriol does *not* provide the cardiac and bone protection that is supplied by the more potent forms of estrogen, an issue of particular concern since Mary's father died of heart disease in his midfifties. However, Mary's cholesterol, blood pressure, triglyceride, and lipid levels all look normal. For now, her cardiac profile indicates that the first steps she could take toward avoiding her family history of heart disease would be to work on some of her lifestyle issues, notably her eating and exercise patterns. And although she is taking micronized natural progesterone to minimize some of her mood swings, it provides the added health benefit of building bone mass, offering her important protection against osteoporosis later in life.

If the trends revealed by the preliminary research on saliva testing continue, and if the early findings and anecdotal examples are borne out by further controlled study, we may find that it is possible to restore a woman's estrogen, progesterone, or other hormone levels to normal physiological ranges with significantly lower dosages of hormone supplements. Currently, if a woman chooses to take HRT, customizing her regimen can sometimes be a hit-or-miss affair. The standardized dosages are either too high for some women and produce unwanted side effects, or else they are too low to adequately relieve symptoms. Saliva testing could allow us to be much more precise in developing individualized treatment plans. It's exciting to think that one day we will stop thinking in "standardized" ways about women's hormonal health.

Another breakthrough that may come about as a result of saliva testing is the ability to measure the effects of plant-based substances, such as soy and black cohosh, on hormone levels (see chapter 7). While these substances have estrogenic properties (they are sometimes referred to as phytoestrogens), we're not sure about their pathways in the body or their effects. Phytoestrogen plants vary tremendously in their potency and in their ability to bind to receptor cells in the body. It may be that in the future saliva testing will provide some of the key answers we're looking for about the therapeutic potential and possible side effects not only of phytoestrogens but what we now call "traditional HRT" as well.

Right now, we don't know all there is to know about measuring hormones through saliva, but this emerging information has certainly commanded my attention. I also appreciate the fact that saliva testing is convenient and private — you do it at home using small plastic containers provided by the laboratory, then mail the containers to the lab for analysis. The lab mails the results to you and your health care provider.

You may be interested in measuring your hormone levels with saliva testing, but your health professional may not yet be familiar with this tool. It is reasonably well accepted among physicians that women's hormone levels vary, so you might approach the discussion from the standpoint that you want information about your baseline levels in order to gather more information about yourself, or to help you decide about any treatment for perimenopausal symptoms. Ideally, baseline hormone testing would be done fairly early on in your perimenopausal transition. Then if you decide to use any intervention to manage your symptoms, follow-up testing is an option to measure your results, using the baseline values as a comparison. As we follow Janice, Sharon, and Mary's progress, we'll be able to assess the extent to which their hormone levels change.

TRUST INTUITION AND TECHNOLOGY

Regardless of whether you use blood or saliva testing to gain more information about where you are in the hormonal landscape, there are two crucial points you should keep in mind about all hormone testing. First and most important, our intuition about our bodies is something we can and need to trust to help us evaluate objective test results. More women than you can imagine tell me, "For a long time, maybe forever, I've known something was going on with my hormones." Second, when it comes to hormone testing, once is not always enough. Sometimes hormone levels need to be assessed again at different times, particularly if a woman is taking HRT. (We'll talk more about HRT in chapter 6.)

Laboratory tests can help us explore and investigate, but they won't provide the final word. Some time ago, I heard a retired physician who was a guest on one of the morning news shows talk about how the field of medicine has changed. "Years ago," he remarked, "we used to listen to what our patients told us. Now it seems we only pay attention to what the lab studies show."

His point really resonated with me, because it seems especially true when assessing women's hormonal changes. Countless women have told me over the years that they intuitively understood that many of their physical and emotional changes were hormonally related. Yet they had trouble finding someone to pay attention to what they were saying and to take them seriously. We need to *listen* to ourselves and to other women, and to use laboratory studies as valuable tools to provide more data about what we know is true. After all, we live in our bodies. Our wisdom about our bodies, combined with appropriate test results, will yield better information than one without the other. Putting the two together is another way of respecting and honoring ourselves.

THE ARC BENDS TOWARD MATURITY

Hormonal shifts and variations appear to "bookend" the beginning and end of our fully fertile years—from our first signs of maturity as young girls, to where we are now, in our forties. During our perimenopausal years, we may be fertile some months (when we do ovulate) but infertile other months (when we don't ovulate). These hormonal fluctuations are similar to those in a young woman who has just started her menstrual cycle but doesn't yet ovulate every month.

Eventually, the ovaries' gradual tapering off of estrogen and progesterone production stops altogether. With estrogen and progesterone no longer stimulating the production and shedding of the uterine lining, menstruation comes to an end. A woman is considered officially "menopausal" when she has not had a menstrual cycle for twelve consecutive months. Reaching this point in her hormonal landscape is usually a decade-long progression of gentle and gradual changes.

Today, women live more than one-third of their lives *after* menopause. We can look at perimenopause, then, as a key threshold, a time for us to give careful consideration to how we live while our reproductive functions change. We can take advantage of the womanly wisdom we have gained in getting to this point in our lives. We can call upon all of our understanding to make this part of our journey authentic, positive, and powerful. As we weigh our options, we need to look at the benefits our hormones provide in preserving our physical and psychological health, and make choices about how to achieve optimum health and vitality when our bodies no longer produce these substances.

Some of us will find that a combination of lifestyle changes and complementary or alternative remedies takes care of the majority of the physical and emotional changes that occur during perimenopause. For others, a different eating plan, a new exercise routine, or vitamin or herb supplementation alone just won't be enough. Those of us who have a family history of heart disease, osteoporosis, breast cancer, or depression face other choices about making the years ahead our healthiest. There is no single path through perimenopause and the years beyond that is right for all women, but we do share a destination—a healthy, productive and fulfilling way of life.

CHAPTER FOUR

Memory, Moods, and Productivity

Around a woman's fortieth birthday she starts hearing jokes and innuendoes—or making them herself—about mood swings, depression, and memory loss. It's not that long ago that the "change of life" was believed to turn women into nasty old crones or dimly aware, befuddled old ladies.

In reality, many of us finally hit our stride in our forties. We advance in our careers, start our own businesses, make a difference in our communities, and usually act as the anchor for our families. All of our talent, skill, and good intentions notwithstanding, we also can find ourselves unexpectedly sidelined by seemingly mysterious changes in our memory, moods, and energy levels. These changes are of varying intensity: for some of us, occasional forgetfulness, transient fatigue, or a "blue" day now and then will be minimally disruptive. But frequent memory lapses, chronic fatigue, and volatile mood changes not only make our days less productive but rack our self-confidence and leave us feeling like we don't recognize ourselves.

For many of us, the timing of these mood changes, memory gaps, and energy shortages couldn't be worse. Of course, there wouldn't be a *favorable* time to blank out in a meeting or squint uncomprehendingly at a spreadsheet as Janice did, but in the midst of a career that is really taking off, sudden holes in memory or difficulty concentrating can threaten the gains you've worked so hard to achieve. Just when you need more energy than ever to move through your busy days, finding that simple tasks require monumental effort is discouraging. Moods that career from anxiety to tearfulness to irritability, often without warning, can rattle your view of yourself and cause your family to tiptoe around you, wondering what's wrong.

Many women in their forties don't connect their experiences with a possible hormonal change. Many worry secretly that they just aren't as sharp as they used to be, or that they just can't cope with life's pressures as effectively anymore. These symptoms — depression, anxiety, irritability, fatigue, mental fuzziness — can also be particularly hard to sort out because they feed on each other. The more tired we are, the harder it is to concentrate during the day, or the more likely it is that we will feel irritable and down. "Am I tired because I lay awake worrying last night? Or am I irritable because I had no sleep? Do I have trouble focusing because I've been feeling depressed?" I talk to many women whose perimenopausal anxiety or depression seems to produce still more worry: "What's going on? Is there something wrong with me? Why am I feeling this way?"

In this chapter I want to unravel the mystery surrounding perimenopausal memory changes, mood swings, and fatigue. We'll take a look at hormonal influences on memory, mood, and productivity, then examine ways to sort out the differences among biological and external variables affecting our recall, outlook, and energy. Most important, we'll look at ways of managing these changes so you can get on with your life with your customary energy, determination, and enthusiasm.

DESPERATELY SEEKING SLEEP

"I don't have *time* to be tired," Colleen burst out in frustration one day in my office. "For me, absolutely the worst part of this time in my life has been the loss of energy. I never wake up feeling like I'm ready to go. I'm in a fog. Then, even though I go to bed early, I don't sleep well. I'm exhausted many days by three in the afternoon. Being tired so much of the time really gets in the way of doing what I want to do."

During perimenopause, sleep, or lack of it, is a big part of the mood swings, mental blurriness, or absentmindedness that can disconcert us. If you lie awake listening to the clock tick or sit in front of the television bleary-eyed, watching your third infomercial at three-thirty A.M., you're not alone. Chances are, thousands of women in their forties are also lying awake, wondering how in the world they're going to think straight, function, and have energy when their day starts in three short hours.

Sleep deprivation caused by perimenopausal insomnia can shorten your temper, drain your energy, and trigger a flood of tears because you're just too tired to deal with anything, from a small inconvenience to a major problem. Night after sleepless night takes its toll, physically and emotionally, leaving you longing for a good night's sleep much as a starving person yearns for food. The relationship between loss of sleep and feeling short-tempered, out of it, or anxious during the day is complex—sleeplessness doesn't directly cause your wavering moods, but it certainly is a major contributing factor.

Humans spend more time sleeping than any other species on earth, yet sleep researchers still don't know exactly why we sleep. While most sleep research has been done on men, one European study revealed that women actually need more sleep than men, up to an hour and a half more per night. Why, then, when we're in our forties, do so many us have trouble getting a decent night's rest?

The reasons are varied, complex, and interrelated. Some women's sleep is disturbed by hot flashes at night, called night sweats. We can wake up soaking and have to change our nightclothes and bedding. By the time we've done all that, we're wide awake.

Surges in follicle-stimulating hormone are linked to hot flashes and night sweats. Remember FSH? This hormone often works overtime during the forties, urging our bodies to release eggs from our ovaries as if to meet a reproductive deadline. Instead of a monthly pulsation of FSH levels, perimenopausal women may have arbitrary spikes in this hormone, which is believed to have a vasodilating effect. FSH opens the capillaries beneath the skin—blood rushes into them, and we heat up.

When an FSH surge occurs at night, we can awaken feeling uncomfortably warm. Some perimenopausal women experience both night sweats and hot flashes during the day—others have only one of these two symptoms, or neither. Researchers still aren't exactly sure why the trigger for night sweats and hot flashes varies from woman to woman.

Another possible culprit in perimenopausal sleep loss is serotonin, the neurotransmitter (brain chemical) that plays a strong role in governing sleep patterns and mood. Estrogen boosts the production of serotonin in the brain, and it may also keep serotonin from being reabsorbed by other cells, so its effects last longer. As our bodies manufacture less estrogen during perimenopause, serotonin may also be in short supply (or it may act for shorter times in the brain), producing wakefulness or restless sleep.

Estrogen's effects on the brain are very similar to the effects of certain antidepressant medications on mood—medications like Prozac, Paxil, and Zoloft also block cells from reabsorbing serotonin. At least one study has shown that estrogen acts more quickly than antidepressants in slowing down serotonin reabsorption. Ironically, some women who take a serotonin-enhancing medication such as Prozac to combat their feelings of depression or anxiety are also battling one of the medication's side effects—insomnia.

The hormone melatonin, produced by the pineal gland in the brain, also strongly influences our sleep and waking cycles. You've probably heard or read about melatonin—it's widely available over the counter and has been alternately called a miracle hormone with anti-aging properties and dismissed as hype.

Here's what we do know about melatonin. Our bodies produce less of it as we get older, and some people find 3 to 5 mg of it very effective in counteracting jet lag (which is really short-term insomnia). As a short-term sleep aid, melatonin may be useful to break the cycle of insomnia, but I'm not comfortable recommending that perimenopausal women use it for long periods of time. My concern is that we run the risk of "programming" our bodies to expect higher-than-normal levels of melatonin so that over time, we could have difficulty sleeping if we haven't taken melatonin. Moreover, some over-the-counter melatonin products contain amounts of this hormone that are significantly higher than what our bodies produce—up to a hundred times the amount. As with any hormone supplement, be it an over-the-counter product or a pharmaceutical-grade medication, the concept of putting a large amount in our bodies isn't one that most of us feel comfortable with.

The good news is that your sleepless nights don't have to go on forever, and you don't have to buy under-eye concealer by the case to hide your dark circles. There are several steps you can take on your own to help regulate your sleep cycle. If night sweats are waking you up, try these simple techniques:

- ✦ Regulate the temperature in your room. Make sure it isn't too hot or cold.
- ✦ Wear lighter nightclothes—thin cotton instead of flannel.
- ✦ Use several light wool or cotton blankets on your bed rather than a heavy comforter. It's easier to pull down one light blanket if you get too warm.
- ✦ Spicy food, caffeine, and alcohol seem to aggravate hot flashes and night sweats in some women. Eat lightly in the evening, and if you've been relying on a glass of wine to help you sleep, try chamomile tea instead.

Maybe you've never had a night sweat but still suffer from sleep disturbances. (That was true in my case.) These sleep tips can make a big difference in the quality of your nights and days:

- ✦ It may sound obvious, but lowering your overall caffeine intake is a starting step toward more restful nights. If you must have caffeine, make sure you don't have any late in the day—in fact, noon is a good cutoff point. After all, if your hormones are changing the way you produce the brain chemicals that help you sleep, you don't need caffeine in the mix to keep you even more wide awake.
- ✦ Make a list of all medications, prescription and over-the-counter, including vitamins and herbs, that you are taking. In some people, insomnia can be a side effect of certain medications. For example, some allergy medications are high in caffeine. Also, vitamin B_6 can interrupt sleep—that's why I always suggest taking

it before noon. Talk with your health care provider or with a knowledgeable pharmacist about all the medications you are taking, to be sure that none of them (alone or as part of an interaction with another substance) is keeping you awake.

+ One of the many payoffs of regular exercise is better sleep. Exercising late in the day, though, can make you feel so wired that you can't fall asleep. If that's true for you, build your exercise into the early part of your day—you'll still reap the sleep benefit. Exercise causes the body to produce endorphins and produces an overall feeling of well-being. One of the residual effects of these endorphins appears to be sounder sleep.

+ Along with your body, your mind also needs to be prepared for sleep. That means taking at least a few minutes to wind down before bedtime. Too often, we try to wring every last minute out of the day, working right up until we collapse into bed. But going to bed abruptly after finishing the last task or chore of the day will mean that your mind keeps going full tilt. Reading, drinking a cup of herb tea, listening to quiet music or a relaxation tape, or taking a warm bath or shower can help relax you before bed.

+ Is your bedroom the at-home equivalent of a noisy hotel room near the elevator or ice machine? Look around your bedroom and see what you can do to make it more comfortable and restful. I know some women who pile their nightstands with unfinished business: bills, lists, work-related documents, and reports. They even keep their laptop computer next to their bed. My recommendation is to keep those types of things in another part of the house. Even if you don't have an office or den, keep your "paper trail" on the kitchen or dining room table, or earmark a spot on a closet shelf. Use your bedroom *only* to rest, and avoid the temptation to make it an office.

+ If outside light or noise gets into your room, think about installing heavier curtains or blinds that close more tightly. Some women object to wearing an eye mask or earplugs—if that's true for you, a portable cassette player with a tape of "white noise" may help lull you to sleep. And I recommend that you look at your bed. Are you sleeping on the same mattress you bought back in the 1970s? Maybe it's time for a new mattress and pillow.

Do yourself the favor of reviewing your sleep habits: your sleep environment, when you go to bed and get up, and what you do, eat, and drink before going to sleep (or before lying awake, if this is the case for you). This is a simple way to start smoothing out edgy, cranky, or depressed days. Sleep won't be an antidote for everything, of course, but if you do clean up what sleep researchers call "sleep hygiene" (your sleep habits) and you're still sleeping poorly, it is a signal that you may need something more.

What might that "something more" be? It may be as simple as taking your calcium supplement (preferably calcium citrate, which is best absorbed) at bedtime. Along with its bone-strengthening properties, calcium seems to have the added benefit of helping women sleep more soundly.

Several herbal preparations may also help you sleep:

+ Extract of valerian root acts as a mild sedative (160 mg taken at bedtime).
+ Kava, a member of the pepper family, can also enhance sleep. The active ingredient in kava is kavalactones. If you choose to take kava, read the label carefully and select a brand that provides a dose of 180 to 210 mg daily of kavalactones. This amount is recommended to achieve kava's sedative effects; the preparation is used in smaller amounts (45 to 70 mg daily) to control anxiety. (See chapter 7 for more on herbal preparations.)

MEMORY BANK

Sleepless nights often dovetail into days when your normal ability to recall simple details seems to elude you. You may leave the house feeling sure you've forgotten something, search over and over for your keys or eyeglasses, or walk into a room without knowing what you wanted to do there. "It came as a real shock to me when I started having trouble remembering things. It was always such a source of pride for me to be well organized and reliable, and suddenly I wasn't anymore," said

Deborah, 45. A couple of years went by before she made the connection between her memory changes and the fact that she was perimenopausal. For her, the lightbulb went on after she visited her sister, who is two years older. "When she picked me up at the airport," she told me, "we spent an hour wandering around the parking lot because she had forgotten where she left the car. She was very irritated and embarrassed at first, but after we went up and down the aisles a few times and kept passing the same cars, none of which was hers, the whole thing started to seem hilarious. We ended up laughing."

Later that evening Deborah and her sister had a serious discussion about forgetfulness. "My sister had talked to her doctor a year earlier, when she first started to feel like she was forgetting more than usual — that's the difference in our personalities. I kept it all to myself and thought I was losing my mind. I wish I had realized sooner what was going on. I never thought about estrogen loss being connected to memory. Even if I had known there was a relationship between those two things, I doubt if I would have thought that hormones could apply in my case — I was only in my early forties."

Researchers are taking a harder look at the connection between hormone levels and brain function, and a key area of interest is the role of estrogen in improving memory and concentration. Estrogen has been found to raise acetylcholine production in the brain — acetylcholine is a chemical that helps us retrieve information stored in the brain. One study of a group of women with Alzheimer's disease showed that estrogen improved their ability to remember and to concentrate. A larger, longer-term study showed that postmenopausal women who took estrogen decreased their risk of developing Alzheimer's disease by half. We're still a long way from being able to claim that estrogen can be used as a medication to enhance memory, but this area of investigation does present hopeful possibilities for Alzheimer's patients as well as women wishing to relieve perimenopausal symptoms.

For many women in their forties, understanding why memory changes occur is more powerful than taking any medication. "It was a big relief to me to realize that I wasn't losing my mind," Deborah said. "I make my lists more detailed now, and if I do forget something, I try not to worry about it."

It's important neither to over- nor underemphasize the role of your female hormones in regulating your ability to remember simple or complicated facts. Yes, declining estrogen levels may certainly have something to do with drawing a blank about a routine matter. But you should also look at how much you expect yourself to keep track of, organize, follow through on, and orchestrate on a given day. There are ways to reduce the overload on your brain: by slowing down, delegating certain things, or deciding that you're just not going to take on as much.

MEMORY ENHANCERS

Along with using detailed lists, calendars, and organizers to stay on top of everything in a given day, some women opt to try herbal preparations to boost their memory and concentration. Janice tried 40 mg of ginkgo biloba three times a day to see if it would help with her feelings of mental fogginess. After two weeks of taking ginkgo, she didn't see any results yet—she still felt muddled at times.

"The other day," she told me, "I was asked a question about one of our contracts in a meeting, something I should have been able to answer in a heartbeat. It wasn't that I couldn't remember the details, but I felt like I couldn't organize a succinct reply quickly enough. When I hesitated, one of my co-workers said 'hello?' really loudly. I was mortified."

I mentioned to Janice that it's not unusual that she wouldn't see immediate results with ginkgo. The studies showing it improves mental concentration are based on twelve weeks' use or more. "That's good to know," Janice said. "I was feeling disappointed, like it wasn't working."

Siberian ginseng (which is different from Panax ginseng, the Chinese or Korean variety) is another herbal remedy that some people believe increases mental alertness. They take it as a root extract three times a day for up to two months, with two to three weeks off between courses. One cautionary note—the quality of ginseng products varies widely. You'll want to find a product that contains 33 percent ethanol extract.

FORGIVE US OUR MEMORY LAPSES

I don't by any means want to suggest that you should live with changes in your ability to recall certain things—an uncomfortable moment like the one Janice had in her meeting isn't something you have to accept. But you can use these episodes to take a look at how much you're doing, and how much information others expect you to have at your disposal at all times.

When Nadine forgot to pick up her 11- and 12-year-old sons from a soccer match, she was horrified and a little frightened. "What will I forget next?" she asked me, sounding almost panicky. In reviewing everything she was doing to perform at her job, shepherd her children around, and maintain her apartment, we agreed that it was entirely likely she *would* forget something because there was too much on her agenda. And while the incident of forgetting her sons had unnerved her terribly, it gave her and her sons a good opportunity to go over, again, their emergency plan: how to use the phone cards they have in their wallets, whom to call if they can't reach her. "They took it for granted that I always show up, which of course I do," she said.

Nadine was willing to take a look at exactly how and where she is "showing up," and to see what she might be able to pare down both at work and at home. I suggested to Janice, too, that she look at what she could simplify. Should anyone else in the meeting, I asked her, have been able to respond to the question she momentarily couldn't answer? "Oh, yes," she said. "There are at least three other people who know these details, including my assistant. It's just that everyone is used to me taking the lead."

Since Janice sat in on the monthly meetings where these questions surfaced, I asked if she could hand off some of the preparation to her assistant. She nodded slowly. "Maybe you can ask her to be ready to respond to certain questions next month," I suggested.

I don't think we consciously or deliberately forget things in our forties, but I do believe some of the lapses are hints that we need to pay attention to. It's as if our bodies were saying to us, "Slow down! The hard drive is full—file some things on disk, and put them away, quick!" Or, if you prefer a more quaint metaphor, "Every inch of the blackboard has been covered — erase part of it to make room for more!"

GUILTY OF DEPRESSION

When Karen started to slide into depression in her midforties, she was afraid to tell anyone about it. "I have no reason to feel depressed," she told me. "My marriage is good, my children are wonderful, and I live in a beautiful home. I have so much to be grateful for, and yet I can't control how depressed I feel. I feel guilty, like I am being self-indulgent, and that I should just snap out of it. I also get very anxious about these feelings, like I'm brooding over inconsequential things. I start worrying that something bad will happen to me or someone in my family and that my nameless worries will become a reality. I can make myself almost crazy."

Depression that hits us in midlife is rarely a matter of self-indulgence, and it's not something we can will ourselves to snap out of. A host of factors can influence depression during perimenopause, and women who become depressed at the time of hormonal fluctuations may be experiencing combined effects. In our forties, physical hormone shifts often go hand in hand with major life events — they really are woven together.

Because she couldn't identify anything going on in her life that could account for her depression, Karen hesitated to seek help. She was concerned that she would be viewed as histrionic, unstable, or a hypochondriac. It had been more than a year since she had a thorough physical exam, so I urged her to see her health care provider for a checkup. "Your emotional health is every bit as important as making sure your body is working properly," I told her. I suggested that she and her provider might investigate the possibility that her depression could be related to hormonal changes. She needed to explore both physical and psychological reasons for her depression, I explained.

We've already met Sharon, whose husband recently faced a very serious illness. Her depression and fatigue were very normal responses to an extremely stressful life event. She worried that if his health were to become very compromised, she wouldn't be able to care for him and their children, the youngest of whom they had adopted from another country only a year and a half earlier.

Sharon confessed that in her low moments, she had begun to doubt the wisdom of adopting their youngest child. "We went through the long, complicated, and expensive process of adopting her because we thought we could provide a loving, stable environment for her," she confided. "I think that we do, but there are days lately when I feel so distracted or depressed, I don't think I do the best job of being her mother."

Distracted, depressed, and overwhelmed in midlife by the demands of a toddler — it's possible that Sharon would have had these feelings even if her situation were not compounded by her husband's health scare. Considering the relationship between her hormonal patterns and what was going on in her world helped her to distinguish between her issues individually so that everything didn't blend together and loom larger than life. Sharon and Karen had very different situations, one more turbulent and the other with an almost enviable stability. Yet both were battling feelings of depression. What's important here is that hormonal variations may certainly be a factor in both cases, and that this component should be neither overlooked nor dismissed.

SUBTLE CONNECTIONS

Not all women become depressed as their estrogen levels decline, so it's impossible to draw a direct connection between perimenopause and depression. But research does show that estrogen has a positive effect on mood. While we can't say estrogen decline *causes* depression, we do know that estrogen's action on the brain involves an interplay with chemicals like serotonin that are believed to be very important in regulating mood. And as we have seen, estrogen's harmonizing with progesterone is also implicated in balancing or unbalancing our moods.

Some women report a perimenopausal mood change that isn't exactly anxiety or depression, but a curious flattening out of their emotions that leaves them wondering where their former energy and joy have gone. Audrey, 44, told me about not only tiredness but about an even more troubling feeling: "You know, sometimes I feel like the energy and excitement I used to have about life just aren't there now. I miss that. I used to be much more vital. Is it my age? Is it because I'm a middle-aged mother? Is it because life's demands are just too much for me to handle? Or is something going on with my hormones?"

Audrey and I reviewed her day-to-day life. The mother of a three-year-old, she is married and works between twenty-five and thirty hours a week. The demands of her work are considerable even though her job is part time, and she finds herself torn between work and the duties of being a mom, with little or no time for herself.

We looked at the potential causes of her fatigue and what she called "lack of excitement about life." Was she getting enough sleep? Was she eating the kinds of foods that would give her energy? Did she have enough help and support in raising her three-year-old son? Did the pressures of her job make it impossible for her to unwind for the rest of the day? When our hormones are fluctuating during perimenopause, our stress level can both influence and be a by-product of these chemical changes. Low progesterone may produce anxious feelings, and our bodies try to mediate the effects of stress by pouring out more adrenaline and cortisol.

After considering these possibilities, we decided that taking a hormone profile would be helpful. With Audrey's health care provider, we agreed to have her saliva tested. The results were revealing: although she was still menstruating regularly and her cycle hadn't changed much, Audrey's estrogen levels were actually quite low. She wasn't off the charts, but she was simply at the very lowest end of the scale, which surprised her physician and me because her cycle was still so regular.

After reviewing the results of the saliva test, we jointly discussed what might be beneficial for Audrey. It appeared that she led a healthy lifestyle and was taking relatively good care of herself. But her hormonal picture did leave something to be desired. We decided to try a one-cycle course on a very low dose of estrogen (0.25 mg Estrace twice a day) and natural micronized progesterone (200 mg daily) to see if she felt better. During the trial cycle, Audrey charted her symptoms so we had an objective record of her mood and energy levels. It didn't take a full month before she called to let me know how she was doing. The changes in the way she felt, as she put it, were "subtle" but "dramatic." "My husband is saying things to me like 'I feel like I have you back,'" she said. "Instead of waking up and wondering how I'm going to make myself get out of bed, I actually look forward to the day."

Audrey is a perfect example of an early-forties woman who doesn't fit any particular mold: a regularly menstruating woman with a very busy lifestyle, who pays attention to diet, rest, and exercise, but whose hormone profile shows that she is very low in one of the most important female hormones.

It's important that you avoid second-guessing yourself during perimenopause. If you have an intuitive sense that something "isn't right" with the way you feel, you have the right to speak out and seek help. You may decide to check your own hormone profile, either through saliva or through blood testing. This information won't provide the final word on why you may feel depressed, anxious, forgetful, or fatigued, but objective data can be useful in adding to the sum of what you know about yourself.

ANXIOUS MOMENTS

Some women have feelings of depression *and* anxiety. Ellen, a 49-year-old mother whose grown child recently left home to work, was one. An active community volunteer, she had a stable marriage and home life. When she came in to see me, she said, "My periods are still pretty regular—the only change is that they're much lighter than they used to be. But my emotions are out of control. I feel like I'm having panic attacks."

Ellen's hormone profile suggested that she was menopausal. (Her estradiol level, when measured with a saliva sample, was less than 1 pg/ml.) However, because she still had a relatively regular menstrual cycle, she assumed, correctly, that she couldn't be menopausal. (Remember that a woman is not considered menopausal until she has stopped menstruating completely.) Ellen was unfamiliar with the term *perimenopause*, so she was unsure of how she should interpret her symptoms. She wondered if she was crazy. Before she came to see me, she had seen a psychiatrist who prescribed Xanax and an ob/gyn who prescribed a low-dose birth control pill after testing her estrogen. Was it confusing? Completely.

Ellen's panic attacks weren't the result of having either too much time on her hands or too much to do. In fact, she seemed quite content with the balance of things in her life before they started. In her case, low progesterone levels may have been the driving force behind the panic. The low-dose birth control pills she was taking may have helped address the estrogen decline. (It's interesting to note that the estrogen in these oral contraceptives is often of a higher amount and greater potency than the estrogen prescribed as part of a hormone replacement therapy regimen specifically for perimenopausal symptoms.) The other important variable in low-dose oral contraceptives is that they contain synthetic progestins. Synthetic progestins suppress the body's production of progesterone. In some women, synthetic progestins greatly worsen anxiety, which may be because their bodies respond poorly to the shortage of the hormone nature intended for them to have.

Ellen had no family history of either heart disease or osteoporosis. She didn't necessarily want to use hormone replacement therapy at this time. Her uterine lining was still being stimulated enough to produce monthly periods. (The estrogen in the oral contraceptives may have had this stimulatory effect.) It seemed appropriate to try progesterone therapy—200 mg of natural micronized progesterone daily for three weeks. Progesterone does not have to be used in conjunction with estrogen, even though estrogen must not be used alone in women who still have a uterus.

Ellen discontinued the birth control pill and felt better within a week. She started using micronized natural progesterone and felt significantly less anxious. This solution may sound too simplistic. But the reality is that in some cases we treat symptoms with different medications and end up treating the side effects of one medication with another drug. In Ellen's case, it would be important to keep the whole picture straight by following up and monitoring her estrogen level. To do this, we would test her estrogen and progesterone levels again in thirty days. This would tell us more about the ratio of estrogen and progesterone in her body and ensure that the dosage of natural progesterone was appropriate for her.

Mary, one of the perimenopausal women we've already met, also chose to try natural progesterone to alleviate her persistent anxiety. I'm not suggesting that natural progesterone is a panacea for anxiety, but I do want to point out that many health providers may not offer it as an option. Although natural progesterone has been used in Europe for decades, it is still something of an "alternative" approach in the United States. More frequently, American women are prescribed an anti-anxiety or antidepressant medication. If you are feeling persistent anxiety or panic attacks, natural progesterone is among the choices you may want to consider.

Why is progesterone often effective in managing feelings of anxiety? While estrogen appears to have an elevating effect on our moods, progesterone seems to calm or relax us—there really is an exquisite balance between these two hormones in our bodies. Produced in massive amounts in pregnant women, progesterone may be the reason why some women feel peaceful and serene when they are expecting. In fact, anti-anxiety medications like Valium act on similar sites in the brain as progesterone. Progesterone is sometimes used to treat PMS, based on the theory that inadequate levels of this hormone in the second half of the menstrual cycle contribute to premenstrual anxiety. An out-of-kilter ratio between estrogen and progesterone may also account in part for anxiety or depression during perimenopause.

I say "in part" because some scientists believe that women who become depressed during perimenopause are predisposed toward this depression for other reasons, and that women with perimenopausal depression are likely to have been depressed *before* their reproductive hormones begin to change. I don't totally agree with this. I see too many women for whom life had been moving along smoothly before they reached the perimenopausal phase, and who then found themselves feeling depressed for the first time.

Sadness and worry in our forties may have a hormonal component, but these feelings can also be heightened by our circumstances. Reaching our forties can have a sobering effect, as we realize we are not immortal. Many women face losses during their forties: their marriage may end, their children leave home, their parents may become ill or die. I don't want to give the impression that perimenopausal depression or anxiety is an "either-or" situation—we can't say that hormones either have everything or nothing to do with the way we feel. We are neither ruled by our hormones nor exempt from their effects. Rather, I'm suggesting that we should look carefully at hormonal influences on our moods and be prepared to take an inventory of other personal issues that can contribute to our feelings of unhappiness or tension.

ANTIDEPRESSANTS IN PERIMENOPAUSE

Too many women, more than I can mention, have told me that while they themselves didn't understand the connection between their mood, memory, and energy changes and their hormonal shifts, their health care providers didn't make this connection either. Many of these women had been diagnosed with depression, and it's true, they *were* depressed. Yet their providers had looked at their feelings of depression (or anxiety, or lack of energy, or sleep disturbances) separately, outside the context of what was going on with their hormones. In many cases, these women left their providers' offices with a prescription for an antidepressant medication.

In recent years new antidepressant medications have come on the market that represent real hope for people with clinical depression. I'm not opposed to antidepressants — they do wonders for many people. But I *am opposed* to overprescribing antidepressants to women whose depression is only one piece of a larger, much more complex picture.

It helps to think through your feelings of depression. Are these feelings new? Do they seem random or are they connected to any life situations that you can identify? Then, if antidepressant medication is offered as an option to you, here are some questions to discuss with your health care provider before you agree to take it:

1. Has a thorough evaluation of my hormone levels been done?
2. Which medication is recommended, and which symptom(s) will it alleviate?
3. Have you prescribed this medication to many women with symptoms like mine, and what have been the results?
4. How soon should I expect relief?
5. How long will I need to take the medication?
6. Are there any side effects I can expect? If so, what are they, and what can I do to minimize them?

7. If this medication does not relieve my symptom(s), what is the next course of action?

Most important, if you are not comfortable taking a particular medication recommended to you, feel free to let your health care provider know. If anything about a medication seems intimidating to you, or if you are unsure of the consequences of starting or stopping it, it's perfectly acceptable, and in fact it's in your best interest, to say, "That's not for me." Antidepressants are not your only choice.

What are your alternatives if you want to get your depression under control but are hesitant about taking Prozac, Zoloft, Paxil, or similar medications? I won't call St. John's wort a "nontraditional" remedy for depression, because although modern health care providers certainly don't routinely recommend it, it has been used for centuries as a healing substance. An extract from this plant can be taken three times a day (300 mg each time) to relieve depression. Michael Murray is a naturopathic physician and expert in herbal medicine whose book, *The Healing Power of Herbs*, is an excellent resource. Dr. Murray recommends these steps to get the most from St. John's wort:

✦ Choose a product that contains 0.3 percent hypericin.

✦ Take St. John's wort with food to avoid gastric upset.

✦ Avoid prolonged exposure to sunlight. St. John's wort has caused sensitivity to sunlight in animals that graze on large amounts of the plant.

Cycles of fatigue, depression, anxiety, or forgetfulness do not have to rule your life in your forties, although these troublesome symptoms can seem to edge out your former energy and zeal. The first step toward gaining renewed energy and a more vibrant outlook is to recognize that there may be a hormonal component in these changes—you are not simply less able to cope or keep up. Second, it's helpful to decide what you want to change, internally and externally, to recapture your physical and spiritual vitality. Our bodies give us the best guidance and the clearest messages when we need more rest, less pressure, more joy, and fewer tasks. Some of the simple lifestyle changes I've discussed here can make a big difference, but real relief will come when you understand that you have the power to bring balance and calm into a life that may have become erratic and hurried.

STRENGTH FROM WITHIN, FROM EACH OTHER

Memory, mood, and energy changes may be hard for you and your health provider to sort out—there aren't any pat, "off the shelf," "one size fits all" answers to these issues, any more than there is a standard prescription for medication that works for everyone. Yet by no means do you have to resign yourself to fatigue, worry, or depression, as if they were an inevitable part of growing older. It's important to keep the big picture in focus as you look not only for the cause but for the best solution to these symptoms. The intricate interplay between your hormones and how you feel, what you remember, and how much verve and energy you have can't be overlooked in your evaluation of what you need to feel healthy and fulfilled. Nor should you underestimate the value of making lifestyle choices that may improve your sleep, jump-start your energy, and restore a sense of peacefulness and contentment.

In all likelihood, you won't find any "outside" solution that will entirely take care of your feelings of anxiety or sadness. No herb, no medication, no lifestyle improvement has as much power as that which you hold within yourself. That's not to say you must call on your own reserves to snap out of what you legitimately feel—you don't have to do it alone.

There is an African folk tale in which women are called upon to bring an enormous and frightening snake back to their chief. (The men, by the way, have already tried without success.) The women are very fearful of the big snake, but the legend has it that "they held on to each other and they were strong." By holding on to each other to conquer their fear, they succeed, bearing the massive snake aloft in their arms. The fearsome snake is presented to the chief, and the women are celebrated for their courage.

The idea of women holding on to each other for strength is a deeply resonant one for us in perimenopause. You may find strength and inspiration by listening to the wisdom of an older woman who has gone through this transition, asking her what it was like for her and what she learned. It can help simply to talk to someone who has been through the transition, gotten to the other side, and has not only survived but in all probability is better and stronger for it.

We can also create new rituals involving women our age who are sharing this transition, putting our own imprint on the ancient and time-honored practice of women gathering together. The possibilities for these rituals are limitless. Whether you favor holding an occasional get-together for tea, participating in a monthly meeting to discuss books or pick stocks, walking with women friends in beautiful places, cooking and sharing a special meal, making a quilt as a group, or participating in a prayer circle, you will come away from these gatherings replenished, sometimes laughing, and always, I think, a little bit more carefree. Far from accepting a fate that would have forties women miserable, tired, and distracted, we can hold on to each other for strength, staking a claim to a decade of strength, vitality, and optimism.

CHAPTER FIVE

Planning Ahead for Healthy Heart, Bones, and Breasts

*O*nly recently has *preparation* become a watchword in women's health. The generations of women who came before us didn't start thinking about steps they could take toward having a healthy pregnancy until they became pregnant. Now, we advocate that women begin to prepare their bodies for pregnancy a full year before they would like to conceive by improving their diet, exercising, and taking essential vitamins. The same is true for perimenopause: whether you are at the beginning, middle, or end of your forties, the time is right to think about making your mature years healthy and enjoyable.

Most women are no strangers to planning ahead for milestones in our lives. We've picked out wedding and bridesmaids' dresses in anticipation of getting married, polished our résumés before graduation, studied the want ads in anticipation of getting a new job, and decorated nurseries while waiting for babies to be born. Perimenopause is another time in our lives when preparation now pays big dividends later.

In this chapter, I'm going to review the healthy steps you can take to protect your heart, bones, and breasts during perimenopause. I'll take you through a *calm* discussion of the risk factors for disease and what you can do to minimize them. Since women are living longer than ever now (our average life expectancy is nearly 80 years) and are in much better health than previous generations, you want to do everything possible to establish good health for yourself in the coming years, judge your risks, and make solid, carefully thought-out choices based on your individual needs.

PROTECTING YOUR HEART

I'm going to start with an overview of how estrogen impacts the heart. Up until the beginning of perimenopause, when our bodies start producing less estrogen, women have a distinct advantage over our male counterparts as far as the health of our hearts is concerned. Women have fewer cardiovascular problems early in life, probably because the "estrogen edge" helps keep our veins and arteries in better shape. But that changes as we get older, when heart disease becomes the leading cause of death among women.

In her book *The Female Heart*, Marianne J. Legato, M.D., observes that by age 60, women's risk of heart disease is equal to men's. After age 65, heart disease kills more women than men — nearly half a million each year. Research data show, and I certainly observe this in my clinic, that the majority of women mistakenly believe that cancer poses a greater threat to their health than heart disease. In reality, heart disease claims more women's lives each year than any other disease, *including breast, ovarian, and lung cancer combined.* I cite this statistic not to sound an alarmist note but to focus on opportunities we have during perimenopause to pay equal attention to our cardiovascular health.

ESTROGEN AND THE HEALTHY HEART

Among the hundreds of beneficial effects that estrogen has in the body, this key hormone protects the heart by keeping the lining of the veins and arteries slippery and free of plaque buildup, so that blood can move freely through them. Plaque (like the plaque that builds up on teeth if we don't brush them) takes the form of granular, sandlike particles, and in our blood these particles can attach themselves to the sides of veins and arteries if those surfaces are rough.

Plaque-filled artery and vein walls are something like a plugged-up garden hose. If you ran chocolate syrup through your garden hose every day, the syrup would eventually stick to the sides and harden. After a while the opening in the hose would be too small to let anything through. In the bloodstream estrogen prevents plaque from getting a stronghold and sticking to vein and artery walls, which then could result in narrower openings that restrict blood flow.

Estrogen also impacts on cholesterol. We've heard the word *cholesterol* for years now, but what exactly is it? It's a waxy, fatlike substance found in the blood. Not all cholesterol is the same, as you may know. "Good" cholesterol is called HDL, and it's considered good because it transports cholesterol and other lipids (fatlike substances) from the body. The "bad" cholesterol is called LDL, and it has a negative impact because it delivers lipids to body tissues.

The ratio between HDL and LDL is extremely important. We want to have a high level of HDL in relation to LDL. A good HDL-to-LDL ratio is 3 to 1, according to Dr. Legato's book, *The Female Heart*. Estrogen helps keep the HDL high and the LDL low.

Your weight, family history, and ethnicity have some bearing on the health of your heart. For example, if your father had a heart attack before age 56 or your mother had a heart attack before age 60, your risk of heart disease increases. Carrying around extra pounds also places you in a higher risk category, particularly if your weight is 20 to 30 percent higher than the acceptable range for your height. If you have a history of heart disease in your family, you have more reason to be concerned about your heart than a friend who doesn't have the same kind of family history.

Mary lost her father to heart disease fifteen years earlier, when he was only 55. A successful businesswoman, she attributes many of her achievements to the work ethic her father demonstrated and to the guidance he gave her when she was first starting out in the work world. Yet when perimenopausal mood changes and loss of libido started to interfere with her life at 42, she hadn't stopped to consider that heart disease could potentially be another part of her father's legacy—it simply hadn't occurred to her.

Mary is certainly not in any immediate danger—her cholesterol, blood pressure, and triglyceride levels are all within normal ranges. But I felt it was essential that Mary take a proactive approach to minimize the possibility of an unwelcome inheritance of heart disease. I reassured her that history wouldn't necessarily repeat itself, but I also reminded her that her choices today about what she ate, how she took care of her body's fitness, and how much stress was a driving force in her life would have a lot to do with her health outcomes in the years ahead.

HRT AND YOUR HEART

Women with a family history of heart disease may find themselves buffeted by conflicting information about hormone replacement therapy and heart protection. We'll talk in more detail about HRT in chapter 6, but I want to emphasize here that when it comes to protecting your heart, HRT needs to be weighed as one of a range of options you have. A family history of heart disease is one factor to consider in evaluating the benefits of HRT—evidence shows that HRT can reduce the incidence of heart disease by as much as 30 to 50 percent. But in our forties the tools at our disposal to strengthen and protect our hearts certainly aren't limited to medication. I prefer to aim for the overall goal of good health and resilience and do what we can do now, on our own, to achieve it without medical intervention.

Perimenopause is a time to begin anew, to make a strong commitment to taking better care of ourselves than we ever have before. A very important aspect of your self-care is paying attention to what your heart is telling you. It's true that men and women who report cardiac symptoms are often treated very differently by the health care system, but it's also true that women themselves often dismiss signals of heart trouble. If you have any concern about a possible cardiac symptom, you owe it to yourself to be sure that this symptom is fully explored. And you may have to be assertive in insisting that it be checked out, if your health care provider seems reluctant to do so or if he or she wants to attribute it to anxiety without any further exploration. In other words, you may have to take the lead in educating your health care provider about the risks of heart disease in women.

The American Heart Association lists these warning signs of a heart attack:

+ Uncomfortable pressure, fullness, squeezing, or pain is felt in the center of the chest, lasting more than a few minutes.
+ The pain may spread to the shoulders, neck, or arms.
+ Chest discomfort with lightheadedness, fainting, sweating, nausea, or shortness of breath may also occur.

If you have pain in your chest radiating into your left arm; a tightness in your chest accompanied by shortness of breath; or palpitations, contact your health care provider *right away*. Note that palpitations can also be a symptom of perimenopause. Some perimenopausal women say their heart pounds abnormally hard or fast when they are having a hot flash, while others have palpitations that are not connected to hot flashes. Again, I want to underscore the importance of not making any assumptions about these symptoms. Talk them over with your health care provider and ask to have the appropriate investigation to rule out a heart problem.

Women who are affected by cardiovascular disease have a less favorable prognosis than men, for a host of reasons. In the past, the medical community tended to interpret danger signs differently for men and women, although this is slowly changing. Still, palpitations in women are frequently attributed to anxiety, while in men they are viewed as a more serious sign of potential heart disease. A more complete diagnostic workup will usually be done on a man who reports chest pain than on a comparable woman. The medical community is beginning to pay closer attention to signs of heart disease in women — a long overdue change that women in our age group can take credit for because we have insisted upon being heard.

If a woman is incorrectly diagnosed as having anxiety, however, when heart disease is the real culprit, her treatment will be delayed or inappropriate. By the time the problem is correctly identified, she will probably have more advanced coronary disease than her male counterpart. Delaying treatment for coronary disease lessens the opportunity for effective intervention. Again, if you experience the warning signs of a heart attack, there are two rules to heed: get medical help immediately, and insist that a heart attack be ruled out. Honoring and respecting yourself means listening to your body when it is talking to you.

The Female Heart cites sobering statistics on women who have heart attacks:

+ Thirty-nine percent of all women heart attack victims will die within the first year of the attack, versus 31 percent of all men.

+ A woman is twice as likely as a man to die within the first sixty days of a heart attack.

+ After a first heart attack, a woman is twice as likely as a man to have a second heart attack.

These statistics can be alarming, especially for those of us whose mothers or fathers have had heart attacks. But you don't have to feel like you may suddenly be blindsided by a heart attack — there is a lot you can do to keep your heart healthy so you don't find yourself facing those post-heart attack odds. For example, smoking not only causes lung cancer and emphysema but also increases the risk of heart attack. You can cut your risk of heart disease by stopping smoking, exercising regularly (women who exercise regularly are three times less likely to have heart disease than those who don't), minimizing your stress level, and paying attention to your diet.

SAME ADVICE, NEW DECADE

"'Exercise. Eat well. Don't smoke.' But I know all that," I can hear some of you objecting. "What's different about that when I'm in my forties than when I was twenty-five or thirty-five?"

Not a thing about the fundamentals of these maxims is new in our forties, I will grant you that. But what should change significantly is the way in which we practice these golden rules, bringing a much more integrated, balanced approach. Eating well is less about being thin and more about strengthening our bodies and giving us energy to step out into our busy days. In our forties we also choose foods that benefit our hearts and bones. The same is true for exercise: the size of your waist is less of a payoff than the relaxed and exhilarated feeling you have after a brisk walk on a beautiful day, and the satisfaction of knowing that you're doing your part to keep your heart and bones working well and to reduce your risk of breast cancer, without medical intervention. Just as our generation of women transformed the experience of childbirth in the late 1960s and early 1970s, we now lead the way in redefining health, giving a uniquely female emphasis to wellness, prevention, and nurturing ourselves.

BUILDING STRONG BONES

Canadian singer kd lang belts out a song about a "big-boned gal" who moves across the dance floor with vigor and joy. Her "big bones" are the essential frame that gives her the power to dance with confidence and enjoyment. You probably think less about your bones than about many other parts of your body unless you've had the painful experience of a fracture: nothing calls attention to the importance of our bones until we're temporarily unable to use some of them.

Ignoring the health of our bones can have serious consequences. Osteoporosis, sometimes called the "silent disease," often exhibits no symptoms, but it insidiously thins and weakens our bones until we suffer a fracture, the first and only sign that our bones were deteriorating. The fact that osteoporosis exhibits no symptoms confuses many women. According to the National Osteoporosis Foundation, women often believe that stiffness, pain, or joint swelling are symptoms of osteoporosis when in fact these symptoms signal arthritis, an entirely separate condition with different causes and treatments. A woman who does not understand the difference between osteoporosis and arthritis may have a false sense of security because the absence of symptoms may make her believe she is not at risk for osteoporosis. Osteoporosis doesn't kill us; it just causes so much misery that it significantly changes our lives.

Bones are living things, constantly absorbing and casting off substances in processes called resorption, when old bone is removed, and formation, when new bone is developed. If you were to look at a cross-section of a bone, say a bone in your wrist, you would see tiny holes, which means that the bone is porous. Osteoporosis affects our bones by making those tiny holes bigger, so that a cross-section of the same wrist bone with osteoporosis would look much like honeycomb. Osteoporosis causes bones to lose mass and density, lessening their strength and their ability to flex. They become brittle and weak and can easily fracture.

We've all heard horrible stories about bone fractures in older women, or perhaps such an incident has occurred in your own family: the woman who turns to put her toothbrush away and falls, breaking her hip in that simple movement. Or the woman who lifts the Thanksgiving turkey from the oven and fractures both wrists, spending the rest of the holiday in the emergency room. One of my patients, Faith, told a particularly heart-rending story about her mother: her osteoporosis was undiagnosed until an exuberant hug from her grandson cracked two of her ribs.

Hearing about Faith's mother reminded me of a dear friend I had when I was in my early twenties, an older woman who was like a second mother to me. At 51, she fell on a patch of ice and broke her wrist. A smoker, she didn't exercise or take calcium. This happened twenty-five years ago, before the word *perimenopause* existed. The rest of her story is one of those "if only" tales. If only someone had recognized that her fracture signaled possible osteoporosis. (The sad irony is that she was married to a physician, and not even he realized that her broken wrist was a red flag.) If only she had been educated about exercise, calcium, the risks of smoking, and HRT. She eventually developed emphysema, suffered spinal fractures, and endured debilitating pain. Finally, when she reached 70, her physician suggested that she consider HRT. If only she had known about her options sooner.

This woman's saga, with all of its "if only" scenarios, is, in one sense, a story of the time in which she lived. What happened to her was tragic and avoidable. If she had been a member of our generation, she might have had more information about her health and might have taken proactive steps to reverse the trend indicated by her broken wrist at 51. Yet even today women of perimenopausal age still may not have access to the information they need to ward off the possibility of developing osteoporosis later in life.

While osteoporosis affects both women and men, women suffer from the disease in greater numbers. It's likely that hormonal influences and exercise and eating patterns combine to contribute to the higher incidence of osteoporosis in women. As young girls, we probably participated in fewer sports or other physical activities than boys. We were the spectators, watching our brothers and male classmates build up their muscles and bones. In people of both sexes, most bone mass is built up in the first thirty years of life, and the bone mass of adults is related to how much weight-bearing activity (running, jumping, and so on) we did before we reached 30. This early bone mass development is a good reason to encourage the children in our lives, boys and girls, to get plenty of physical exercise and to make exercise part of our own "playing" with our daughters, sons, nieces, and nephews.

The more bone mass we have, the longer it takes to lose it. Women have smaller body frames than men, with 25 to 30 percent less bone mass, which may also be why women develop osteoporosis earlier in life and more often than men. In addition, the aftermath of "career dieting" can be reduced bone density, particularly if we haven't been careful about getting enough calcium.

Our hormones play a key role in keeping our bones healthy:

+ Estrogen promotes the absorption of calcium.
+ Estrogen acts on cells in the bones called *osteoclasts*, which dissolve old bone. The hormone inhibits these cells from dissolving bone at an excessive rate.
+ Progesterone has a bone-building effect, acting on *osteoblasts*, or cells that form new bones.
+ The hormone testosterone (usually mentioned in connection with perimenopause only for boosting libido) also builds bone by stimulating osteoblasts.

It is estimated that women lose 50 percent of the bone mass that we are going to lose in our entire lifetime during the first seven years of estrogen depletion. Clearly, estrogen decline is only one factor in this scenario—progesterone and testosterone also play roles in bone build-up and breakdown. But since we don't know exactly when we start to lose estrogen, we really can't pinpoint the beginning of this bone mass loss. We do know, however, that preventive measures to minimize bone loss can start today.

These statistics from *The Osteoporosis Handbook* made me sit up and take notice:

- In the United States, more than 1 million fractures result from osteoporosis every year.

- Half of the people who could walk unaided before a hip fracture cannot do so afterward.

- Every year 50,000 deaths result from hip fractures. Deaths occur because of blood clots, pneumonia, and other complications.

- Fifty-four percent of women who are 50 today are expected to have some type of fracture due to osteoporosis during their lifetime.

The bones most affected by osteoporosis are those in our wrists, spinal column (vertebrae), and hips. When the bones in the spine become weak, we can develop spinal fractures, which are extremely painful. You probably have seen women with dowager's humps—they are hunched over with a distinct curve at the top of their spines. The next time you are in a public place with a lot of people, take a look around—chances are you'll see an older woman with this stooped appearance. She has probably sustained breaks in several of her vertebrae, one on top of another, which ultimately led not only to her shorter stature but also to her prominent hump at the top of her back.

As is the case with heart disease, family history plays a role in women's personal risk for osteoporosis. If your mother broke her wrist when she was in her fifties, had a vertebral (spinal) fracture in her sixties, or broke her hip as she aged, you are more likely to develop osteoporosis than the daughter of a woman who experienced none of these things.

Some medical experts say that if you have a family history of osteoporosis, hormone replacement therapy is a must for you. A calm, calculated assessment of your risks is in order, along with a thoughtful discussion between you and your health care provider.

There are several ways to determine whether you are losing bone too quickly. One way is to have a DEXA, a diagnostic procedure that measures the density of your bones.

DEXA FACTS

+ *DEXA* stands for "dual energy X-ray absorptiometry."

+ DEXA is a low-dose X-ray, usually done on the wrist, hip, and a section of the spine.

+ DEXA is done with a special X-ray machine, not the regular kind used to X-ray a broken bone.

+ Not all health care facilities have DEXA machines.

+ A DEXA costs between $150 and $200. Not all insurance companies cover this cost. You may be able to make a successful case by pointing out that the cost of the test is far below the cost of hospitalization for a fracture.

You may want to talk with your health care provider about having a DEXA. If your DEXA test results reveal that you are losing bone mass early and rapidly, you can take several concrete measures to stop bone deterioration. We'll discuss those later in this chapter. But you might want to have a DEXA done now, then follow it up with another DEXA in a year.

DEXA results are used by women and their health care providers to:

+ assess baseline bone density, particularly if the woman has a family history of osteoporosis.

+ evaluate whether medication is needed to arrest bone loss or to build back new bone.

+ determine if a treatment for bone loss or restoration is effective.

Bone loss can also be detected through a laboratory test that measures bone fragments (deoxypyridinoline) that are released into the bloodstream and then excreted into urine. A special urine test indicates the rate of bone resorption (bone loss) and thereby assesses the condition of your bones.

When Mary and I reviewed her health profile and family history, she mentioned that a friend of hers, also in her forties, had had a DEXA. "Should I have one done too?" she asked.

I told her that measuring bone density or bone loss isn't necessarily routine when we're in our forties. Her decision on whether to have a

DEXA or the urine test, I said, would depend on why she wanted the information and how she intended to use it. If bone loss was suspected, either because of a fracture or a very low estrogen level, a bone study might provide important additional information.

Right then there were no immediate red flags that said Mary should have a bone study. But her low estrogen and progesterone levels (both may affect bone loss), combined with the fact that she rarely exercised, raised her own concern that her bones could be thinning. She did take calcium to supplement a diet that wasn't always the healthiest. Now it was as if the attention she had focused on her perimenopausal mood changes and her drop in sex drive had also piqued her curiosity about her overall health.

Since she had had her hormones measured with the simple saliva test, she said, the urine test to measure bone loss appealed to her. She could do it the same way—at home, without missing time at the office. I said I appreciated her wanting to save time, but that time spent on her health would be an investment she could easily justify. I wasn't necessarily advocating that she have the DEXA, which requires a visit to a medical facility, instead of the urine test; I just wanted to reinforce the point that we are never "too busy" to monitor our health.

The results of Mary's urine test showed that the rate of her bone breakdown was not excessive—something she was relieved to hear. Her bones didn't show any damage that she needed to try to reverse. So she could look at the gradual lifestyle changes she was making in her eating and exercise routines as a means of maintaining good health.

Faith also had the urine test to detect bone loss because we had more to be concerned about in her case. If you recall, her mother had severe osteoporosis and suffered a broken rib. In addition, Faith's saliva test for progesterone and estradiol levels showed that she was very deficient in both hormones. The results of her urine test for bone breakdown weren't what we would have preferred. Normal values are between 3 and 6.5, and anything above 6.5 indicates abnormally rapid bone breakdown. At age 40, Faith's results were right at 6.5, the very highest we would want them to be. She looked stricken as we talked about her test results. Almost in a whisper she asked, "Will I have to be careful about having my son hug me, just like my mother?"

Not in the least, I assured her. "There's plenty we can do right now, not only to slow the rate of bone breakdown but to build back some of the bone you've lost." I told her about some self-care options she could begin that day: extra calcium, more weight-bearing exercise, follow-up testing in a month, and if bone breakdown continued to accelerate, natural progesterone. She asked me for an extra copy of these steps. "I want to send it to my mother," she said. "I don't know if she's been made aware of all of these things." Faith felt encouraged about her ability to strengthen her body, and she was also going to network within her own family to be sure her mother had all the information and options she did.

BREAST HEALTH IN OUR FORTIES

The specter of breast cancer strikes at some of our greatest fears and vulnerabilities, threatening our femininity, sexuality, and ability to nurture. As one woman said, "Breast cancer hits us where we live." I want to address the issue of breast cancer here in a way that helps us move from anxiety to action. It isn't always easy or straightforward, because there are no clear-cut, tidy answers that can put our concerns about breast cancer to rest. But we can better understand our risks and use the same solid reasoning that we use to make decisions about other aspects of our health. In that way we can feel like we are doing all that is currently possible to minimize the probability of developing breast cancer in our forties.

LOOKING AT THE NUMBERS

The information about breast cancer is hard to sort out. On the one hand we hear scary statistics about the rising incidence of the disease and warnings that one in eight women will develop it. Yet we also hear that breast cancer is being detected earlier and that the cure rate is increasing.

Let's pause, take a deep, calming breath, and look at what these numbers really mean. First, the one-in-eight figure does *not* mean that if you're sitting with a group of eight friends, one of you will develop breast cancer. That's because not all women of all ages are equally subject to this "one in eight" risk. A woman's risk of breast cancer changes as she ages: before age 40, her chance of getting breast cancer within the next ten years is 1 in 233, according to the American Cancer Society. Between 40 and 50, she has a 1-in-65 chance. The risk increases as she ages: after 50 her probability of developing breast cancer within the next ten years is 1 in 41, and after age 60, 1 in 29. The majority of women who develop breast cancer do so after age 65. These numbers do not provide reassurance, but they provide perspective.

Other factors besides age are considered in assessing a woman's risk of developing breast cancer:

+ Number of first-degree relatives who have had breast cancer (sister, mother, grandmother, aunt)
+ Age at first period (menarche)
+ Age at first childbirth
+ Number of breast biopsies that show abnormal tissue

Early menarche, delayed childbearing, and late menopause are all associated with an elevated risk of breast cancer. But even these risk factors are not precise indicators; they merely help to determine the probability that a woman will develop breast cancer. The reality is that the majority of all breast cancers appear in women who have *no* risk factors.

The presence of the breast cancer genes (BRCA1 and BRCA2), which were identified in 1994, also indicates a higher risk of breast cancer among certain women. When a copy of either gene is damaged or flawed, cancerous cells in the breast can develop—approximately 10 percent of breast cancers are caused by defective BRCA1 or BRCA2 genes. The breast cancer genes have many mutations, and as yet no uniform guidelines are in place to advise a woman about treatment and prognosis if genetic testing reveals that she carries a damaged gene.

BREAST CANCER RATES

After climbing by an alarming four percent per year from 1982 to 1987, the incidence of breast cancer appears to have stabilized in recent years, neither dropping nor rising dramatically. Each year more than 184,000 cases will be diagnosed, and nearly 45,000 women will lose their lives to breast cancer. Some researchers and advocates refer to the incidence of breast cancer as an epidemic. Regardless of how we view the incidence of breast cancer, it feels like an epidemic to every woman who has been touched by the disease, either personally or through someone she loves.

I was recently reminded of how vulnerable we feel in the face of breast cancer when Sharon came in for a follow-up visit. Her perimenopausal symptoms of fatigue and depression had been compounded by the fact that her husband was recovering from a serious illness. Now she learned that her husband's mother, to whom she was very close, had had a recurrence of breast cancer several years after her original diagnosis. "I'm just numb," Sharon said. "It seems like too much for our family to take."

Numb. Too much to take. Those were some of my own feelings a few years ago, when my routine mammogram showed a possible abnormality. When I heard my doctor say, "We're going to have to do a biopsy," the room suddenly got very small, as if I were watching from a great, great distance, and my blood seemed to pound in my ears. So pure was my panic that I almost couldn't drive home. I am deeply thankful that the breast tissue in question turned out to be benign in my case, but I will never forget those terrified few days, and I hope that if I ever have to repeat them, I will find the strength I need.

KNOWING YOUR BODY

The issue of breast cancer becomes even more highly charged for women in their forties who are considering hormone replacement therapy to relieve perimenopausal symptoms or for potential heart and bone protection. The research data are contradictory, with some studies showing a strong relationship between HRT and breast cancer and others finding that HRT has no effect on incidence of the disease. Chapter 6 discusses breast cancer and HRT more thoroughly, but before we get to that point, I want to outline the proactive steps you can take, giving yourself a measure of control even when you cannot precisely predict your risk of this disease and in spite of information that is often difficult to interpret.

You know your own body better than anyone, and you need to be as familiar with your breasts as you are with every other part of yourself. If you're not yet in the habit of examining your breasts every month, make a commitment to start this month. You can hang a reminder in the shower—some health care facilities provide waterproof instruction cards when women come in for mammograms. The best time to examine your breasts is two to three days after your period ends, when your breasts are less likely to be tender. Women who no longer have regular periods can mark their calendars for the first of every month to remind themselves to examine their breasts. The goal of practicing regular breast self-exams (BSEs) is, again, to become more familiar with your breasts and to learn to recognize changes in them. It's important to remember that most often, breast changes are normal and benign.

It may help you to feel more comfortable about examining your breasts if your health care provider goes over the procedure with you. He or she can point out areas in your breast that feel firmer than others, building confidence in your own ability to recognize changes in your breast tissue. In addition, your health care provider should examine your breasts yearly when you have your regular physical and Pap smear.

BREAST SCREENING WITH MAMMOGRAPHY

Having a baseline mammogram (an X-ray of the breasts) provides an important picture of your breasts that will be compared with mammograms you have later on. Mammography can detect a breast cancer as small as a grain of sand, long before it could be felt by hand during a regular breast self-examination. And when breast cancer is detected early, it can often be treated more successfully. If you haven't yet had a mammogram, today is the day to call for an appointment.

In spite of evidence showing that early detection of breast cancer leads to better outcomes, research shows that as many as one-third of women over 40 have not had a mammogram. In my practice, I often encounter women who put off this important health screening. "I'm afraid the mammogram will show something suspicious," said 41-year-old Lee. "There's a part of me, and I know it's irrational, that doesn't want to know if I have breast cancer." Joanne claimed she was hesitant not because of the possible results of a mammography but because the thought of having her breasts compressed on the X-ray plate made her shudder. If you've had feelings like Lee or Joanne, let me tell you how we worked through both of their concerns.

Lee and I talked about her fear. "First of all," I told her, "it's not irrational at all. It's a very real response. But it might help you to acknowledge that fear and ask for some support. Can you schedule a mammogram with a sister or friend so you can both have one the same day? It's always reassuring to have company when you're doing something for the first time."

Lee shifted in her chair, but then she sat up a little straighter and nodded. "I do have a friend who would go with me," she said. I mentioned to Lee that if her friend had a different doctor or insurance plan and couldn't go to the same facility for her mammogram, she and her friend could agree to go with each other on different days.

Lee and I also talked more about her view of mammography. "Maybe we can shift around your thinking," I suggested. "Rather than 'finding out if you have breast cancer,' what you're actually doing is taking care of this part of your body. It's a way of telling yourself, 'I deserve to be healthy.' Why don't you and your friend have breakfast or lunch on the day of your mammograms? You can celebrate a lot of things — the fact that you're both taking good care of yourselves."

For most of her primary care, Lee sees a nurse practitioner; she resolved to call her the next day to schedule a mammogram. I recommended that Lee ask her nurse practitioner for specifics about the process: "You'll want to know who reads your mammogram, who will notify you of the results, and by when. The more you know going in, the more comfortable you'll be able to feel."

I handed Lee the piece of paper where I had written the questions she might want to ask her nurse practitioner. She took it and nodded again. "I'll call my friend when I get home to ask her to go with me," she said. Our discussion hadn't completely taken away Lee's nervousness, but I could tell that she was taking a big step toward confronting something that frightened her.

Joanne was concerned about the pressure or possible pain during mammography, so we talked about what she could do to overcome her concern. "Most women don't find the procedure painful," I said, "but the time when you schedule your mammogram can make a difference. It helps to schedule it after your menstrual cycle, when your breasts won't be tender." (Joanne's cycles are still fairly regular. But some perimenopausal women whose menstrual cycles have become erratic can't always predict when their breasts won't be tender. If this is true for you, make your best estimate. If it turns out that your cycle changes and your breasts are sore on the day of your appointment, you can reschedule it. Just be sure not to put your appointment off for too long.)

I also reminded Joanne that she was in charge of the procedure. "If the position of your breast on the X-ray plate is too uncomfortable," I suggested, "ask the mammography technician to adjust it." As I did with Lee, I suggested that Joanne go with a friend, and that she too ask about the process in advance.

Many women, like Lee and Joanne, have their first mammograms in their forties. The American Cancer Society and the American Medical Association recommend that women over 40 have a mammogram every year. After equivocating for a time, the National Institutes of Health has joined in this recommendation. You may want to talk with your health care provider about your age, overall health, and family history to come to an agreement about the most appropriate and comfortable mammogram schedule for you. If insurance coverage for mammograms is a concern for you, check with a hospital in your community or your local branch of the American Cancer Society. Hospitals and community health organizations sometimes offer free or low-cost mammograms to women who need them.

THE PERSONAL IS POLITICAL

It's true that breast self-exams and mammograms are not fail-safe methods for detecting breast cancer. We even hear grumbling that mammography can lead to "unnecessary biopsies," an argument that always amazes me. None of us would choose an unnecessary biopsy, but neither would we choose an unnecessary death from breast cancer that a biopsy might have prevented. I feel very strongly that even though they are imperfect, we need to avail ourselves of the screening procedures that we have now. At the same time, we don't have to accept that that's all there is. We can continue to push for development of more exact screening measures and for more research on breast cancer causes and treatments. We can stress the urgency of our concern by writing, calling, or e-mailing elected representatives to press them to direct funds toward these ends, and by supporting breast cancer advocacy organizations of our choice. It is women our age who are completely rewriting the rules about how health care is delivered. This impact is very visible in the momentum that the fight against breast cancer has gained in the last decade. We can't completely predict or control our risk of developing this disease, but we can at least feel satisfied that we've done everything within our power not only to protect our own health but that of women who will follow us into perimenopause.

LIFESTYLE CHANGES

ANSWERS ON YOUR PLATE

Clearly, my discussions with Faith, Mary, and Lee had different points of emphasis. Faith was frightened about ending up frail at an early age like her mother, Mary had just begun to realize that her father's early death from heart disease potentially impacted her health, and Lee's worry about breast cancer had produced a form of inertia when it came to getting a mammogram. Yet to all three of these women, as well as to dozens of women *who have no family history of heart disease, osteoporosis, or breast cancer,* I made some basic recommendations about packing more health into each bite they take.

- ✦ Consider the source—of protein, that is. Not only does excess meat in your diet drive up your cholesterol level, but the digestive process necessary to break down meat causes your body to use additional calcium. If you regularly consume meat in servings larger than a deck of cards or the palm of your hand, give some serious thought to switching to other protein sources like soy, beans, and some low-fat dairy products. Soy in particular has been shown to help lower cholesterol.
- ✦ Don't go cold turkey (no pun intended). I'm an advocate of gradual changes. If you're accustomed to eating meat daily or several times a week, choose a different protein source one meal at a time, once a week, until you've discovered several alternative dishes you enjoy.

◆ Omega-3 fatty acids, which are found in mackerel, herring, tuna, sardines, salmon, and shellfish, may play a role in preventing heart disease. Like meat, fish is animal protein — less preferable than plant-based sources of protein — but on the occasions when you do enjoy fish, choose one that provides these essential fatty acids.

◆ *Low-fat* or *fat-free* doesn't always mean "healthy." It amuses me to see bags of jelly beans and other candy labeled "fat free!" in the grocery. Monitoring how much fat is in your food is a good idea, but don't go overboard with counting fat grams either. A low-fat diet can help to keep cholesterol at a healthy level, and there is some suggestion, although the research is not conclusive, that reducing dietary fat may also lower breast cancer risk.

◆ Eat two to three calcium-rich foods at every meal. Calcium is essential to keep bones strong. Among your high-calcium choices are many foods that are heart-enhancing as well as bone-strengthening — low-fat, high-fiber beans, collard greens, and spinach, for example.

CALCIUM-RICH FOODS

FOOD	AMOUNT	CALCIUM CONTENT
YOGURT	1 CUP	415 MG
MILK	1 CUP SKIM, LOW-FAT, WHOLE	300 MG
CHEESE	1 OZ. CHEDDAR, SWISS, OR MOZZARELLA	200–270 MG
COTTAGE CHEESE	1 CUP	155 MG
RICOTTA CHEESE	½ CUP	335 MG
MACARONI AND CHEESE	1 CUP	360 MG
ICE CREAM	1 CUP	175 MG
COLLARD GREENS	1 CUP	355 MG
SPINACH	2 CUPS RAW	110 MG
BEANS	1 CUP NAVY OR SOY, COOKED	95–130 MG
SALMON	3 OZ. CANNED, WITH BONES	165 MG

- Moderate your caffeine intake. Taking more than 400 mg of caffeine a day (two large mugs of drip coffee would put you at the limit) will cause your body to excrete calcium in your urine.

- Take 1500 mg of calcium (preferably calcium citrate) each day to keep your bones strong.

- A word of caution about calcium: more isn't better. More than 3000 to 4000 mg calcium per day is difficult for your body to absorb and can cause kidney stones.

- Vitamin D (400 to 800 I.U. per day) helps the body to use calcium properly. Sunshine is the best source of vitamin D, but as we get older our bodies are less able to absorb it.

- Take 100 to 400 I.U. of vitamin E daily. The Harvard Nurses' Health Study showed this may reduce heart attack risk by at least 40 percent.

- Stress reduction is an important part of keeping your heart healthy. Certain herbs such as kava, valerian, and ginseng have a calming effect. See chapter 7 for more on complementary approaches to health.

- Celebrate wisely. Like caffeine, excess alcohol (more than two drinks daily) can rid your body of the calcium you need. Drinking a moderate amount of alcohol may have some protective effects against heart disease, osteoporosis, and possibly breast cancer. However, there's no standard definition of "moderate" drinking, so I'd recommend that you think of alcohol as something to enjoy sparingly on special occasions.

- Check your medicine cabinet. Some medications hasten bone loss, including drugs commonly used to treat arthritis, asthma, lupus, thyroid problems, and epilepsy, as well as certain antacids that contain aluminum. Ask your health care provider if any medication prescribed to you puts you more at risk for bone loss. And read over-the-counter medication labels carefully—some are high in caffeine.

UP IN SMOKE

Smoking substantially increases the risk of heart and lung disease, osteoporosis, and breast cancer. It's not exactly new information, but many women aren't aware that women who smoke reach menopause sooner. Their bodies stop producing estrogen at an earlier age, robbing their heart and bones of estrogen's protective effects. And even during their fully fertile years, smokers appear to benefit less from estrogen's influence. It's as if smoking counteracts the positive consequences of estrogen.

Smoking among women, particularly women under 25, is on the rise. When I was a teenager, my mother smoked, and so did most of my friends' mothers. Not only do we owe it to ourselves to take good care of our bodies during our perimenopausal years, but we have an added obligation to act as positive role models for young women. If you smoke, I strongly encourage you to find a way, any way, to begin the process of stopping. I've been there myself, and I won't say it was easy or that I didn't miss smoking, but in the sixteen years since I had my last cigarette, I've never regretted my decision to get rid of the habit.

I lit my first cigarette at 17, hoping to fit in with my peers, trying to look grown up, and perhaps unconsciously imitating my mother. For fourteen years I smoked cigarettes regularly, although I stopped during both of my pregnancies, only to start again after my sons were born.

When my sons were 10 and 12, they started lecturing me about the dangers of smoking. (The tobacco education program in their school was very effective.) They also applied that irrefutable brand of logic kids use: "If candy bars are bad for us and cigarettes are bad for you, every time you have a cigarette, we should be able to have a candy bar, right?"

Being a mother has always been my most important and challenging job. I realized that I owed it to my sons to set a better example and to take better care of myself as well. I made a commitment to myself to go cold turkey. Quitting was tough—I chewed nails off, and maybe a few people's heads. Nor did I quit smoking all at once. In fact, I slipped on occasion in the beginning and had a few cigarettes, but afterward I had a headache, bad breath, and the horrible feeling that I could go back to a destructive habit. Today when I pull out old photos and come across one of me with a cigarette in my hand, I'm thankful I was able to change that part of my history.

Women in our age group also have the opportunity to help change the history of any young women we know who may be furtively smoking those first few cigarettes. Warnings about addiction, lung cancer, and emphysema may not sink in, but some young women may be willing to hear you talk about the fact that you respect, rely on, and take care of your body, which is why you don't smoke. The message that you consider yourself too worthwhile to smoke may not produce an immediate behavioral change, but it will plant a seed that may be acted on later.

WE MOVE TOWARD GOOD HEALTH

One of the kindest things you can do for your body is, quite simply, to move it around. Chapter 8 talks more about choosing an exercise routine that works for you, but here I'll mention some basics about types of movement that provide multiple benefits: less stress, cardiovascular conditioning, more bone strength, and lowered risk of breast cancer.

Yoga is an ideal exercise for forties women for a host of reasons: it tones up our muscles and calms us down. We can do it when and where we like, and we don't have to buy any equipment, shoes, or outfits. Another beautiful aspect of yoga is that it is a gentle way to begin moving if you're unaccustomed to exercise. More advanced yoga exercises and poses are suitable for women who regularly exercise. Alternating a more rigorous and jarring form of exercise like running with the soothing and calming stretches involved in yoga is an excellent way to bring balance to an exercise routine. Some yoga poses are weight-bearing — that's the type of exercise you need to do regularly in order to build bone strength. (Weight-bearing exercise simply means that the weight of your body is supported by your bones.)

Walking is another integrated form of exercise that builds your bones, gets your heart pumping, and can also give you a stress-free break from your hectic pace. The act of walking around, either alone or with someone whose company you enjoy, is a conscious way to break away from the pattern of rushing around. You might be surprised at what you notice, as Mary was. The executive who was an avowed nonexerciser, Mary had agreed to hand off some of her phone calls late in the day to her assistant so she could take a short walk. "I was very uncomfortable at first," she said. "I'm just not used to having nothing in my hands. I'm always holding the phone, or the steering wheel of my car, or my briefcase, or the reports I'm reviewing, or I'm pounding the keyboard on my computer. It felt strangely nerve-racking at first to be walking around empty-handed. I felt like I was wasting time."

To her credit, Mary didn't give up walking twice a week. "I didn't want to carry hand weights, so I bought a set of 'stress balls' that fit in the palm of your hand. They're made of soft material that you squeeze. Depending on what my day has been like, I either press them gently or try to pulverize them." A normally serious person, Mary suddenly laughed.

In our forties, exercise doesn't have to be about doing bouncing routines to thumping music in a communal room. Some women are combining their exercise routines with an expression of their spirituality, borrowing from ancient traditions where women gave thanks together for water, sun, good crops, and other gifts from the earth. Today a group of women I know who are members of a synagogue regularly gather outside to exercise and pray together. Reaching for the sky, one participant described the gathering as a "way to send prayers directly up to God." She added, "Exercising and praying at the same time reminds me to be thankful for my body, that it's healthy and strong." Ecclesiastical dance brings movement into some masses or church services, using the body to offer praise and thanks for mysteries and miracles that are, perhaps, beyond words.

MORE THAN SELF-HELP

Many women are unsure about how to evaluate the benefits of their self-care program — how to know if their exercise, eating habits, and stress-reduction techniques are providing adequate protection against heart disease, osteoporosis, and breast cancer. Here again, no single answer works for all women; and no single line says, "If you cross this point, you need more medical intervention than self-care can offer."

But there are some general guidelines you can keep in mind and discuss with your health care provider. When I am working with a woman in her forties who is attempting to improve her health, these are the warning signals we look for together, particularly if she has a family history of heart disease or osteoporosis. The presence of these signals suggests that medical intervention may be necessary.

High cholesterol. A cholesterol level above 240 mg/dl that does not respond to increased soy in the diet, lower fat intake, more exercise, and stress reduction for three months may indicate a risk for heart disease. For a woman who fits this profile, I would look carefully at hormone replacement therapy as an option. As we'll discuss in more detail in chapter 6, HRT sharply reduces the risk of heart disease.

Bone loss. Rapid bone loss, evidenced by a urine test result over 6.5, or bone density significantly below normal range, as indicated by a DEXA, could indicate osteoporosis. Options for managing bone loss include:

- ✦ Natural progesterone therapy. When combined with a regimen that includes magnesium, calcium, vitamin D, and ascorbic acid (vitamin C), natural progesterone appears to have properties that can turn around bone loss. This is a very noninvasive first step. Because progesterone, estrogen, and testosterone all work in concert to prevent bone breakdown and promote new bone formation, these hormones are sometimes used together in an HRT regimen aimed at preventing osteoporosis. When the primary goal is to reduce bone loss, I usually begin with progesterone only and evaluate the results before adding other hormones.

- ✦ Calcitonin, an "antiresorptive" agent. Recent research shows that calcitonin taken *with* calcium provides better bone protection than calcitonin alone. Calcitonin is a very expensive drug, and it may produce side effects such as nausea, flushing, or a skin rash.

- ✦ Fosamax, a nonhormonal drug used to arrest bone loss. The long-term effects of Fosamax have not yet been studied.

Possible future drug treatments for osteoporosis include:

- ✦ Ipriflavone, a soy derivative used in Italy and Japan although not yet in the United States.

- ✦ A new category of medications called SERMs, or selective estrogen receptor modulators. It appears that SERMs may have the ability to provide estrogenlike protection of the heart and bones, yet block estrogen's effects in the breasts and uterus. Sometimes referred to as "designer estrogens," SERMs such as raloxifene, droloxifene, and idoxifene are coming under closer scrutiny by researchers who are investigating possible alternatives to HRT. Raloxifene has been approved by the FDA for prevention of osteoporosis. SERMs are not without side effects of their own, however. They may increase hot flashes and elevate the risk of developing blood clots in the legs. The term "designer estrogen" is good sound bite, but we're a long way from having all the clinical data on SERMs.

In looking at therapies to reduce perimenopausal symptoms, lower cholesterol, or improve bone strength, it's important to guard against the mentality that we can just swallow a pill to "fix" a certain situation, whether that pill is an herb, a vitamin, or a potent drug. I view anything we put into our bodies as a way of complementing or even bolstering the effects of our own self-care. Medication doesn't absolve us of responsibility toward ourselves — if anything, we need to increase our resolve to take better care of ourselves so we can use medication for the shortest time possible.

ACTION REPLACES ANXIETY

Some of the risk factors for heart disease, osteoporosis, and breast cancer are out of our control. You can't change your family history or undo what you did in the past that may not have been the greatest for your health. But you also don't have to feel anxious or threatened, as if you're playing some kind of roulette where you either will or won't be diagnosed with one of these conditions. You have a great deal of control over your odds for positive health outcomes and a long and fulfilling life, and there is power in actually *enjoying* the things you do to stay healthy in your forties.

Taking charge of your health is a way of saying you refuse to go away and let aging take its course. You are insisting that you will move through perimenopause and beyond with a body that expresses robust health, strength on the inside, and vigor on the outside — the ultimate in female sensuousness.

CHAPTER SIX

Hormone Replacement Therapy: Facts About Your Choices

Not long ago I stood in line at the grocery store reading magazine covers. One said, "Estrogen, the hormone of youth!" while the cover directly below it said, "Breast cancer: Is estrogen the villain?" No wonder the issue of hormone replacement therapy seems scary, and even a little crazy, at times.

Newspapers and magazines are filled with articles on the risks of breast and uterine cancer, heart disease, and osteoporosis and how they may be related to HRT. These articles often spell out breaking developments — and provide conflicting information. One article presents HRT as a cause of disease, while another sees it as a preventive measure. Many women tell me they've simply stopped reading these articles. These are intelligent women who are committed to taking care of themselves, but the contradictions in the news stories about HRT leave them feeling confused or frightened or both.

In this chapter, I'd like all of us to take a collective deep breath. Now that we've taken a look at some of the risk factors for heart disease, osteoporosis, and breast cancer, let's take a *calm* look at some basic facts about HRT. In addition to answers to pressing questions about its risks and benefits, many women need fundamental information about *which* hormones are part of an HRT regimen, *where* they come from, *what* they're made of, and *how* they're taken. It's important that we know these basic facts before we begin our discussion of the risks and benefits of HRT.

The purpose of this chapter is *not* to convince you that you should or shouldn't use HRT. Rather, it will give you (1) a better basic understanding of what HRT involves, and (2) a clearer perspective on how your own personal situation fits with this information.

TAKING A CLOSER LOOK

Gail had this to say about the array of confusing information about hormone replacement therapy: "I've attended a half-day workshop on menopause and visited a specialist twice. The specialist patiently explained all the various functions and definitions of the hormones, but I still seem to have a major mental block. Will someone please tell me exactly which hormone does what in a way I can understand and remember?"

The hormone charts on pages 101 and 102 are an answer to Gail and many others like her who have asked me for the same thing: a way to simplify and sort out HRT information. HRT can be a bewildering topic, and I don't intend to gloss over its complexities. But based on questions I hear again and again from women trying to get a handle on HRT, these charts are designed as a road map to lead you to a greater understanding. Their purpose is to:

+ describe the "family" of estrogens: estradiol, estrone, and estriol
+ show that some commercially prepared forms of estrogen match the estrogens produced by the body and are thus considered "natural"
+ clarify the distinctions between synthetic progestins and natural progesterone
+ provide a reference for brand names. When you hear a term like Premarin or Provera, you can find it and pinpoint what it is.

HORMONE OPTIONS: AN OVERVIEW

HORMONE CATEGORY	TYPE	BRAND	FORMS	DOSAGE RANGES
ESTROGEN	ESTRADIOL: A POTENT FORM OF ESTROGEN MADE BY THE OVARIES BEFORE MENOPAUSE	ESTRACE	ORAL TABLET VAGINAL CREAM	0.5–2.0 MG/DAY 0.1 MG/GM (STRENGTH) 2.0–4.0 GM/DAY
		ALORA CLIMARA ESTRADERM FEMPATCH VIVELLE	TRANSDERMAL SKIN PATCH	0.05–0.1 MG/DAY 0.05–0.1 MG/DAY 0.05–0.1 MG/DAY 0.025 MG/DAY 0.05–0.1 MG/DAY
		ESTRING	VAGINAL RING	2.0 MG RELEASED OVER 90 DAYS
		NO BRAND NAME — MUST BE COMPOUNDED BY A PHARMACIST	SKIN CREAM OR GEL	0.05–0.1 MG/GM PER DAY
	ESTRONE: THE PREDOMINANT FORM OF ESTROGEN SYNTHESIZED IN FAT CELLS AFTER MENOPAUSE	OGEN*	ORAL TABLET VAGINAL CREAM	0.625–1.5 MG/DAY 1.5 MG/GM (STRENGTH) 2.0–4.0 GM/DAY
		ORTHO-EST*	ORAL TABLET	0.625–1.25 MG/DAY
	ESTRIOL: THE "WEAK" ESTROGEN, PRODUCED BY THE PLACENTA DURING PREGNANCY; ALSO CONVERTED FROM ESTRONE IN THE LIVER IN SMALL AMOUNTS	NO BRAND NAME — MUST BE COMPOUNDED BY A PHARMACIST	ORAL CAPSULE VAGINAL SUPPOSITORIES VAGINAL CREAM TOPICAL SKIN CREAM OR GEL	1.0–4.0 MG/DAY 0.5–2.0 MG, 2 TO 3 TIMES PER WEEK 0.5–2.0 MG/GM 2 TO 3 TIMES PER WEEK 0.05 TO 0.5 MG/GM PER DAY
CONJUGATED ESTROGENS	CONJUGATED ESTROGENS CONTAIN ESTRONE COMBINED WITH A NUMBER OF OTHER ESTROGENS, SOME OF WHICH ARE UNIQUE TO HORSES	PREMARIN	ORAL TABLET VAGINAL CREAM	0.3 MG–1.25 MG/DAY 0.625 MG/GM (STRENGTH) 0.5–2.0 GM/DAY

*These contain estropipate, a derivative of estrone.

SOURCE: MADISON PHARMACY ASSOCIATES.

		PREMPHASE**	ORAL TABLET	TABLETS CONTAIN 0.625 MG CONJUGATED ESTROGENS AND 5.0 MG PROVERA
		PREMPRO**	ORAL TABLET	TABLETS CONTAIN 0.625 MG CONJUGATED ESTROGENS AND 2.5 MG CYCRIN
PROGES-TERONE	SYNTHETIC PROGESTIN	PROVERA CYCRIN	ORAL TABLET	2.5–10 MG/DAY
	NATURAL PROGESTERONE — CHEMICALLY IDENTICAL TO THE HORMONE PRODUCED BY A WOMAN'S BODY	NO BRAND NAME — MUST BE COMPOUNDED BY A PHARMACIST	EVEN-RELEASE MICRONIZED TABLET	200–600 MG/DAY
			MICRONIZED ORAL CAPSULE	200–600 MG/DAY
			VAGINAL SUPPOSITORIES	200–800 MG/DAY
			RECTAL SUSPENSION	200–800 MG/DAY
			TOPICAL SKIN CREAM, GEL, OR LOTION	10–30 MG/DAY
			SUBLINGUAL TABLET	25–200 MG/DAY
			INJECTION	50–100 MG/DAY
		CRINONE	VAGINAL CREAM	45–90 MG/GM PER DAY

**Combination of conjugated estrogens and a synthetic progestin.

You can also refer to these charts as questions come up for you about perimenopausal symptoms, possible relief with hormones, and potential side effects.

LANGUAGE BARRIERS

First of all, *hormone replacement therapy* is a term that confuses many of us. "Hormone replacement therapy? Does that mean estrogen?" is a question I still hear. The answer is yes and no. Yes, HRT includes estrogen. No, not estrogen alone, unless your uterus has been removed by a hysterectomy. Even if your uterus has been removed, you and your health care provider may decide that estrogen *and* other hormones are necessary.

A typical HRT regimen includes:

+ a type of estrogen

+ a type of progesterone, either natural progesterone or one of the synthetic progestins

+ if needed, an androgen such as testosterone (see chapter 10)

History accounts for some of the confusion between "hormone replacement" and what was once called "estrogen replacement." In the 1960s and early 1970s, estrogen was prescribed *by itself* to women who had perimenopausal symptoms. In fact, just about every woman who complained of a hot flash was put on estrogen replacement therapy. Estrogen taken alone, without natural progesterone or a synthetic progestin, is called *unopposed* estrogen replacement therapy.

Prescribing unopposed estrogen replacement therapy became a routine practice, until an alarming trend started to emerge in the early 1970s: more women taking estrogen were developing uterine abnormalities. Something clearly was wrong.

Estrogen was identified as the culprit, and it was discovered that estrogen *alone* can stimulate the growth of irregular or even precancerous cells in the uterus. Without progesterone, estrogen causes the uterine lining (endometrium) to build up instead of sloughing regularly. The cells become increasingly crowded and may become misshapen or malformed. Cell changes could result that are potentially dangerous, possibly leading to cancerous conditions.

The discovery of the link between estrogen-only regimens and increased risk of uterine cancer set off widespread alarm. In an abrupt reversal of the promise that estrogen would keep them forever young, women were taken off estrogen en masse. In my view, this was regrettable for three reasons. First, many women really benefited from estrogen. Second, in many cases estrogen therapy was stopped before medical professionals understood that the missing piece of the puzzle was progesterone. Third, anxiety and confusing information about HRT and cancer persist today, even though we now know that a *combination* of estrogen and progesterone mirrors the body's natural balance and avoids estrogen-only promotion of irregular uterine cell growth.

Today HRT is different from the estrogen-only approach of the 1960s and early 1970s. For one thing, estrogen dosages, both in HRT regimens and in oral contraceptives, are significantly lower. For another, estrogen is now combined with natural progesterone (or a synthetic progestin) for women who still have their uterus intact. While the estrogen causes the uterine lining to thicken, the progesterone ensures that the lining is regularly sloughed in the form of a menstrual flow.

(A note here for women who have had a hysterectomy and therefore do not have a uterus. Estrogen alone poses no risk of uterine cancer after hysterectomy because there is no uterine lining to be overstimulated. However, some women who have had hysterectomies still choose to take estrogen *with* natural progesterone because natural progesterone has bone-building properties and can also have a calming effect on mood.)

HORMONES

NATURAL VERSUS SYNTHETIC

The word *natural* can be tricky to interpret when we're talking about HRT. When we say a hormone is "natural," we mean it is chemically identical to the hormone produced in the body. Natural hormones are also referred to as "bioidentical" hormones. A synthetic hormone (Provera, for example, which is medroxyprogesterone acetate, a type of synthetic progestin) has a slightly different chemical structure from the progesterone produced by our bodies. Progesterone receptor cells in our bodies will recognize synthetic progestins, but natural progesterone and synthetic progestins act differently in the body and produce different effects on progesterone receptor sites. Natural progesterone molecules fit *exactly* into progesterone receptor cells.

The distinction between "natural" and "synthetic" is very important. First, I want to point out that we're not saying here that "natural" is good and "synthetic" is bad. Not at all. But it's important to understand that natural and synthetic hormones have very specific effects on the body, and that these effects are different. There are appropriate uses for both natural and synthetic hormones, but they should not be considered interchangeable. For instance, some women have trouble tolerating synthetic progestins, whether they take them as part of an HRT regimen or in an oral contraceptive, finding that they produce unwelcome side effects. Some women say they feel weepy, irritable, and bloated when taking a medication containing a synthetic progestin. For these women, natural progesterone is an option to consider.

Second, once women are clear about the differences between natural progesterone and synthetic progestins, lots of them want to know about "natural" estrogen. Many women are surprised to learn that some commercially prepared estrogens match the effects of the estrogens produced by the body and so are considered natural. They are chemically identical to estrogens produced by the body and will affect estrogen receptor cells in the same way. Meanwhile Premarin, which contains certain types of estrogen that are unique to horses, is not considered a natural form of estrogen. Remember, it is the chemical structure of a hormone, not its source, that determines if it is natural or synthetic. A natural hormone may be developed in the laboratory using pharmaceutical-grade products.

Third, the word *natural* is sometimes used pretty loosely. Some herbal preparations claim to be natural remedies for symptoms of perimenopause or premenstrual syndrome. They may be marketed as phytoestrogens or wild yam cream and be plant- or herb-based. If you choose to try one of these preparations, find out all you can about what it contains. It's wise to let your health care provider know what you're using and how much.

WHERE DO HORMONES COME FROM?

The most commonly prescribed estrogen, Premarin, is derived in part from the urine of pregnant horses. Premarin contains a combination of estrone, which a woman's body produces, and other estrogens that are unique to horses. In women, estrone is metabolized in the body's fat tissues. Another commonly prescribed form of estrogen is Estrace (estradiol). Produced by the ovaries in fully fertile females, estradiol is made from a soy base when commercially prepared.

Laboratory synthesis is used to develop synthetic progestins, such as Provera. Natural progesterone is derived from an extract of soybeans or yams and must be compounded by a pharmacist—it is not made in mass quantities and is not widely available. "Can't I just eat lots of soy products and yams?" Gail asked me. I explained that neither soybeans nor yams can be converted directly by our bodies into progesterone. So while these foods are low-fat and nutritious, loading our plates with them won't change our hormone levels. Still, eating soy foods does produce an estrogenlike effect that many women report helpful in managing their perimenopausal symptoms. Some women are also confused about "wild yam cream," which is sold over the counter as a remedy for premenstrual syndrome or perimenopause. Our bodies can't convert wild yam extract into progesterone.

WHICH HORMONES ARE RIGHT FOR ME?

Just as all women have different perimenopausal experiences, no set recipe or formula for HRT works for all women. Actually, quite the opposite is true, and there are variations and options we all need to understand. But the most commonly prescribed HRT regimen includes estrogen, usually Premarin, and one of the synthetic progestins, such as Provera. You may have even heard this combination cavalierly referred to as "Prem and Pro" or "a P&P cocktail."

In the mid- to late 1970s, following the discovery that estrogen alone was dangerous for women who still had a uterus, medical professionals began to add progesterone to women's HRT regimens. Provera, which is medroxyprogesterone acetate, was the usual choice. Physicians correctly assumed that Provera would protect a woman's uterus from irregular cell growth.

Today more prescriptions are written for Premarin than for any other medication in the United States, and Provera is among the top twenty of all medications prescribed. This may be because some physicians become very familiar with certain medications and feel comfortable prescribing them exclusively. Where HRT is concerned, it's important to understand that standardization isn't possible. There are alternatives you need to know about, and in many instances you may be the one educating your health care provider about alternatives. The estrogen and synthetic progestin combination of Premarin and Provera may be a suitable prescription for some women but for many it is not.

I see many women who do not respond well to synthetic progestins such as Provera. Some of the side effects include weight gain, mood swings, headaches, and insomnia. In fact, many women tell me that they discontinued HRT because they didn't like the way they felt when they took Provera, but they feel fine on estrogen alone. Other women I encounter don't do well on Premarin; it may be that the horse estrogens contained in Premarin are poorly tolerated.

In fact, Carmen told me she simply stopped taking Provera and continued with estrogen alone without consulting her health care provider. "I couldn't tolerate Provera's side effects," she said. "It made me feel like I had PMS twenty-four hours a day, seven days a week." I was very alarmed and told Carmen that because she still has her uterus, taking estrogen alone increases her risk of uterine cancer. Since Provera was producing unwanted side effects, I advised Carmen to talk with her health care provider about using an alternative, such as natural progesterone.

Carmen's intuition about her body's inability to tolerate synthetic progestins was right, but it is not advisable to make a change in any HRT regimen without talking it over with your health care provider. After our discussion, Carmen spoke with her provider about natural progesterone. After he read the PEPI trial results I faxed to him (a comprehensive research project that showed the benefits of natural micronized progesterone), he was willing to prescribe it for Carmen, although he hadn't used it with other patients before. Carmen started taking 200 mg of natural micronized progesterone daily in lieu of the synthetic progestin. Four days later I got a phone call from her. "I can't believe it, but I feel like a completely different person. I'm not nearly as irritable, and the waistband of my pants isn't cutting into my skin — I'm not so bloated." The switch produced results that seemed remarkable to Carmen, but in fact I observe similar effects on a regular basis. Women who were ready to give up and stop taking HRT altogether often respond beautifully to a change from a synthetic progestin to natural micronized progesterone.

PATIENT COMPLIANCE

It's estimated that up to 75 percent of women who are prescribed HRT do not take it for the amount of time their health care provider has recommended. This noncompliance statistic doesn't surprise me in the least. Probably two things are going on here: (1) women are being prescribed HRT regimens that are inappropriate for them, and (2) if they experience side effects, no one is taking the time to explain their options or to work with them carefully to arrive at the appropriate medication and dosage level.

I'm not fond of the term *noncompliance* because it suggests that patients should all be good, take their pellets as instructed, and run through their mazes on command like trained mice. To me, women's unwillingness to stick with an HRT regimen that makes them feel ill serves as an important wake-up call to the medical community and to drug manufacturers. We're slowly seeing more awareness of other options: natural hormones, a combination of self-care with medication, and herbal remedies.

Yet other women feel very hopeless after they stop taking HRT, particularly if they don't know other choices are open to them. Isabel tried HRT for six months, dutifully taking her Premarin and Provera daily. She had decided to take HRT in the first place because her hot flashes and palpitations had become very uncomfortable, and she often felt unaccountably depressed. As a result of HRT, "my hot flashes did improve, but my moods were just terrible. I felt even more depressed than I was before I started taking hormones, and I also had horrible irritability. My teeth were on edge every day."

On her forty-ninth birthday, Isabel abruptly stopped taking Premarin and Provera. "I decided to give myself a present. I just decided I wasn't going to feel this way," she said. She felt good about her decision for a few days, but after two weeks she came to see me because she was still struggling with mood changes and she also developed vaginal dryness and burning. "HRT didn't work for me," she told me. "I don't know what to do now. I feel better than I did when I was taking the Premarin and Provera, but I'm unwilling to feel this way for the rest of my life."

I asked Isabel if she had talked with the health care provider who had prescribed Premarin and Provera. She had. "My doctor wasn't disturbed when I told her I had quit taking the HRT. She told me to come in for another appointment. I asked her what else we might try, and she didn't say much. She said, 'Maybe HRT just isn't for you.'"

As Isabel and I talked more, I explained that HRT doesn't mean just one standardized prescription that either does or doesn't "work." When I suggested that she consider a combination of natural progesterone and a different form of estrogen, she looked doubtful. "I'm kind of gun-shy about taking anything else right now. I feel like I want to clear out my system."

"That's fine," I told her. I recommended that she give herself a break for a couple more weeks, and in the meantime I suggested she try some soy foods (they contain phytoestrogens that are helpful in relieving some perimenopausal symptoms) and use a vaginal lubricant. She was willing to have me call her doctor to talk about natural hormone options, and she said she would call me to check in the following week.

THE FORGOTTEN ESTROGEN

The other "different form of estrogen" that I mentioned to Isabel, and that I would be discussing with her doctor, is estriol. Estriol is sometimes called the "forgotten" estrogen because its use is less widespread. It is also known as the "weak" estrogen because it is less potent than the two other types of estrogen produced by the body, estradiol and estrone. Although estriol is available over the counter in Europe, American health care providers are generally less familiar with it than other types of estrogen.

Estriol helps with perimenopausal symptoms such as urine leakage, vaginal dryness, and hot flashes, but it has little or no effect on the heart or bones. Estriol also does *not* act on the breasts or the lining of the uterus, which means that unlike estradiol and estrone, it can be taken alone, without progesterone or a synthetic progestin. It is available in capsule, cream, and vaginal suppository form.

Some women who have used estriol have told me that they think their mood is improved, which is one of the reasons I thought it might be appropriate for Isabel. While there's no study yet to document improved mood with estriol, anecdotal evidence is sometimes an important beginning that leads to a larger investigation. In Isabel's case her depression seemed to lift.

Estriol and natural progesterone were certainly helpful in turning Mary's situation around. She originally came to me for help because anxiety and irritability were causing problems for her in her high-pressure job, and she felt that her relationship with her fiancé was suffering because she had lost interest in sex for no apparent reason. She was now taking 200 mg of natural micronized progesterone daily and using a 0.5 mg suppository of estriol twice a week. After four weeks on this regimen, she came to see me.

Mary always looks very put together when I see her—it's clear that she pays a lot of attention to her clothes and grooming. But she looked especially good the day she came in for the follow-up visit, and it may have been that she looked *happier*. "My moods are much different," she exclaimed. "My job is still the same pressure cooker, but I don't have that out-of-control feeling that I can't handle it."

In addition to taking natural progesterone and estriol, Mary was now walking three times a week after work. "I've started to look forward to those walks," she said enthusiastically. "I leave the office a little earlier—it's really a nice break for me." She also reported that her sex drive had improved. She and her fiancé spent a weekend away earlier in the month and truly enjoyed each other's company. "The bed and breakfast was very romantic, and so were we," she said, smiling. But she grew serious for a moment and said, "It could be that I was able to enjoy having sex because I didn't feel as wound up and stressed out as I had been feeling for weeks. I can't exactly say my sex drive is higher, but I know I feel more relaxed, and that makes a difference."

Mary's observation was very astute. Our perimenopausal symptoms are often intertwined, and relieving one set of symptoms, in her case anxiety and irritability, sometimes has an ancillary effect in relieving others, such as loss of libido. Her modest exercise program had also helped.

OTHER HRT ISSUES

PILL, PATCH, OR CREAM?

If, like Mary, you decide to try HRT to relieve specific perimenopausal symptoms and/or to protect your heart and bones, you can choose from different forms of administration. Women who prefer swallowing a pill have that option for estrogen, synthetic progestins, and oral micronized natural progesterone. "It's easier for me to remember to take pills," said Nicki. "I take my estrogen and progesterone in the morning, when I take my vitamin." If you're taking HRT in oral form, the time of day you choose is up to you. Morning, noon, or evening is fine, as long as you keep the same routine and don't vary it by taking HRT one day in the morning, the next in the evening, and so on.

When you are deciding which form of HRT to try, convenience is certainly important, but it's just one factor to consider. Your decision is best made when it is based on the symptoms you most want to manage, and the level of protection you want to give your heart and bones. After that, convenience and cost may come into consideration.

For instance, estrogen is also available as a skin patch. Some women appreciate the convenience of applying the skin patch and going about their business. The patch also provides the advantage of continuous, even delivery of estrogen. But because the patch releases the hormone into the bloodstream, it bypasses the liver. That means that the patch provides the same bone protection as oral estrogen, but it may not provide as much protection against heart disease.

Some women who suffer from headaches during perimenopause benefit from using a skin patch. Experts believe that perimenopausal headaches are related less to the *amount* of hormones our bodies produce than to the *fluctuations* in these hormones. It may be that the steady delivery of estrogen through the patch levels out the fluctuations, thus helping to relieve headaches.

Estrogen skin patches are now available in several dosage strengths—another hopeful sign that we are moving away from the notion that "one size fits all" when it comes to HRT. Another reminder about the skin patch: you still need to remember to take your progesterone in whatever form you choose; tablet, suppository, or cream.

Estrogen can also be delivered vaginally, either through a vaginal cream or through a vaginal ring inserted somewhat like a diaphragm and left in for ninety days.

Estradiol, estrone, estriol, and natural progesterone are also available in cream form. There is some suggestion that estriol and natural progesterone may provide perimenopausal symptom relief in significantly lower doses in cream form than in oral forms. What's still not known is how much hormone cream is needed to provide heart and bone protection. Women who currently do not have to be concerned about bone loss or cardiovascular disease but who want to manage mood swings, vaginal dryness, hot flashes, or stress incontinence may be good candidates for natural hormone creams. These relatively new developments continue to build our knowledge about HRT options and raise questions that need further exploration. Before you try taking any hormone in cream form, though, be sure you know exactly how much of the hormone is in the cream, and exactly how many milligrams of the medication you will receive when you use the cream. It's best to work with a knowledgeable pharmacist and a reputable supplier of hormone creams (see appendix B).

A natural hormone cream seemed like a good option for Sharon, who had begun six weeks earlier with a self-care program that included increasing the amount of soy in her diet, balancing her exercise routine with yoga to reduce her stress, and taking a vitamin supplement with B_6. But her home situation had recently become more complicated, and she felt increasingly anxious. Soon after her husband's illness, her husband's mother faced a recurrence of breast cancer. Sharon's three children also required a steady supply of her time and energy.

"I'm just not sure I can do all of this," Sharon said, her eyes filling with tears. "I can't even sleep at night, I'm so nervous." For Sharon, "all of this" is considerable: supporting her husband as he continues his recovery, caring for her 11-, 9-, and 3-year-old children, and wanting to be able to respond to her mother-in-law's needs.

For some women with Sharon's symptoms, I might recommend natural micronized progesterone in oral form. But Sharon had already made it clear in our earlier visits that she preferred not to take medication if at all possible, and she very definitely did not want to be on HRT. I suggested that she consider natural progesterone cream, which she could rub into her hands twice daily. "Progesterone cream is medication, but at a very low dose and taken in the least invasive way," I pointed out. "If you decide to try it, you could start with 10 mg a day. Many women find that a small amount of natural progesterone helps with anxiety and irritability, and it can be an excellent alternative to other medications that are often prescribed to relieve anxiety."

We talked about the fact that natural progesterone cream would not be an antidote for the understandable anxiety she was feeling as a result of the very stressful and demanding life events she was facing. "But it just might give you a little extra help, and you need that now," I suggested.

Sharon did decide to try natural progesterone cream for one month. We contacted her health care provider to obtain the prescription, which she then had compounded by a pharmacist. (A prescription hormone cream can be compounded to meet your specific needs. You know exactly how much hormone you're getting, and prescription creams often cost less than creams you can buy over the counter. Many insurance plans will cover the cost of prescription hormone creams.)

I talked with Sharon ten days after she started using the cream. "Oh, I still have plenty of anxious moments, but I'm not quite as overwhelmed," she told me. "Between the yoga class I started, the deep breathing, and the progesterone cream, I can feel a difference."

WHAT DAY IS IT?

A perimenopausal woman on HRT who needs to know what day it is isn't necessarily having a memory lapse. She may be on a *cyclic* HRT regimen, in which the hormones are taken only on certain days. Specifically, on a cyclic HRT regimen, she takes estrogen for twenty-five days, and natural progesterone or a synthetic progestin for twelve days. If both hormones are stopped, she may have bleeding like a period as her body "withdraws" from the hormones. If you and your health care provider decide that a cyclic HRT regimen is appropriate for you, you can work together to determine the best cyclic schedule.

The other method of administering HRT is called *continuous* HRT. In a continuous regimen, estrogen and natural progesterone or a synthetic progestin are taken daily, all month long. With continuous HRT there is no "withdrawal" bleeding, although it may take a woman's body one to three months to adjust to the regimen and to stop break-through bleeding completely. Many women experience fewer side effects with continuous HRT.

RISKS AND BENEFITS

For some of us, the risks of HRT may outweigh its benefits. Women who have had these conditions should be carefully evaluated before HRT begins:

+ breast, uterine or other cancer stimulated by estrogen
+ a family history of estrogen-dependent cancers
+ abnormal vaginal bleeding
+ chronic liver disease
+ blood clots in the legs or lungs

The research on HRT and breast cancer is contradictory. Some studies have shown that HRT is *not* associated with an increase in the disease, but other data link HRT (both estrogen alone and estrogen and synthetic progestins combined) with a greater risk of breast cancer when taken for five years or more. The Harvard Nurses' Health Study is often cited as showing that HRT raises breast cancer risk by 30 to 40 percent when taken for five years or more, and presents an even higher risk for older women. For some women, even a slight risk of breast cancer is unacceptable — Sharon felt that way, particularly since her mother-in-law was struggling with breast cancer. While she had no direct family history, seeing her mother-in-law's situation made her feel very wary of anything that could increase her own risk of developing the disease. Other women decide that HRT's potential benefits for them today outweigh the risks, particularly when their personal risk of heart disease is much greater than their risk of breast cancer. These women, like all of us, need to take care of their breast health by scheduling regular mammograms and examining their breasts every month.

There isn't a single process to arrive at a decision about HRT, and unfortunately we don't have neat answers to the question about breast cancer risk. It will probably be many more years before enough rigorously controlled long-term studies on HRT have been done to tell us everything we want to know. Until then, some women will give HRT a wide berth, preferring to rely on nondrug remedies to keep their symptoms under control. Others will choose HRT, feel well when they are taking it, and be comfortable that, for them, the advantages outweigh the drawbacks. Each choice is personal — no blanket decision will apply across the board. Whatever you decide about HRT, you need to feel that you have had an honest dialogue with a health care provider who knows your situation, and who is willing to seek out the latest research and information about new HRT products as they become available and provide that information to you. Most of all, your decision needs to be made in the spirit of partnership with a professional who listens to and respects your views about your own health.

PROTECTION AGAINST CANCER

We hear plenty about HRT's potential carcinogenic effects, but very little about its possible protective effect against colon cancer. There is some evidence that HRT significantly lowers women's risk of developing and dying from colon cancer. Researchers don't know what mechanism estrogen uses — it may be that it protects the colon lining, reduces certain acids that may promote cancer, or actually inhibits growth of cancer cells in the colon. More research is needed, but the preliminary studies, which showed a 50 percent reduction in risk for women on HRT, are promising.

MANAGING HRT SIDE EFFECTS

Isabel, who considered stopping HRT a birthday gift to herself, is an example of a woman on HRT for whom the "cure was worse than the disease." Her situation doesn't have to be yours. When an HRT regimen isn't relieving your symptoms or is making you feel worse, it's clearly not working. Then you and your health care provider will need to do some adjusting: you may have to change medications, switch to a different form of administration, or take less or more of a hormone.

"I'm fat since I started HRT," Laura stated flatly. "I was never slender to start with, but now I've gone from a size ten to a twelve, and I'm barely fitting into those."

Weight gain can be an unwanted companion of HRT, as the estrogen component of the regimen seems to slow down our ability to burn body fat. Laura's concerns about her weight echo those of many women who are considering HRT. I explained to her that because our basal metabolic rate decreases during our perimenopausal years, it takes our bodies longer to burn the calories that we ingest, whether or not we're on HRT.

Because Laura's uterus was intact, her HRT regimen included a synthetic progestin, to prevent estrogen from stimulating abnormal cells in the uterus. One side effect of the synthetic progestin that Laura was taking can be weight gain. The *Physicians' Desk Reference* (PDR), commonly used by physicians as a source of product information about drugs, says that among the potential reactions to Provera are "fluid retention" and "weight change (increase or decrease)."

Taking HRT doesn't have to mean an automatic weight gain. Laura and I discussed the importance of choosing foods wisely and the benefits of getting enough exercise. Then we identified three options for adjusting her HRT:

+ First, we would talk with her health care provider about switching her from synthetic progestin to micronized natural progesterone. If, after two to three weeks on this regimen, her weight gain, bloating, or both were still problematic, we'd go to the next step.

+ Step two would be to change the type of estrogen she was taking. Laura was currently taking Premarin, which contains estrone and other estrogens that are unique to horses and that may have had a role in her weight gain. Changing to Estrace, which is estradiol, could help. Again, I recommended evaluating this regimen after two to three weeks.

✦ If there were still no improvement in the weight problem, the third step would be to lower the dosage of Estrace. Sometimes a smaller dosage of estrogen can provide the protection we want without contributing to weight gain.

DOSAGE ISSUES

ADJUSTING AN HRT REGIMEN

It used to be that a standard HRT prescription included a uniform number of milligrams of estrogen and synthetic progestin or natural progesterone. But we know now that dosages need to be tailored much more precisely to meet a woman's individual needs. You'll notice that I suggested changing only one thing at a time about Laura's HRT regimen. That would allow Laura and her health care provider to isolate which change provided the most benefit. The same step-by-step change was made for Rhonda, who had been stable on an HRT regimen of oral estrogen and natural progesterone for months, only to experience a sudden recurrence of her headaches and hot flashes. She recently had had a gastrointestinal upset, and together with her health provider, we concluded that this episode might have temporarily affected her ability to absorb the oral hormones. She switched to the estrogen patch for one cycle and felt the difference almost immediately—her symptoms were greatly alleviated.

"How much estrogen or progesterone do I need? What dosage should I be taking?" Women who are considering HRT are often confused about dosages, and understandably so. Most often, they worry that taking too much estrogen, even when combined with natural progesterone or a synthetic progestin, will raise their risk of breast or uterine cancer. We often tend to believe that one prescription, whether it's for perimenopausal symptoms or anything else, is the final word—now we should feel better. We hope the medication will take care of whatever is bothering us, and we're disappointed if it does not. But there's no pat answer to questions about HRT dosages, or at least no way to say that x mg is always appropriate. The chart on pages 101 to 102 shows common dosage ranges. Arriving at the most appropriate HRT prescription may take some work and perseverance on the part of both you and your health care provider. I'm not talking about an extended trial-and-error experiment while your symptoms continue unabated, but a careful evaluation of what you need.

Many perimenopausal women choose to begin with the lowest possible dosages of HRT, adjusting them upward as needed to provide symptom relief. A conservative, low-dose approach is often adequate for perimenopausal women who are still producing some hormones. The lower dosages can offer symptom relief without exposing them to hormone levels that are too high.

While you are taking HRT, it's important to assess your hormone levels through blood or saliva testing to be sure that the amount circulating in the body closely approximates the amount that would be there if your body were still producing all that it needs. The amount of medication required to achieve these levels varies from woman to woman.

In general, circulating estradiol levels of 50 to 60 pg/ml (in blood) are the minimum necessary to avoid bone loss and changes in sexual function. To maintain energy and avoid changes in mood, memory, and sleep patterns, target estradiol levels need to be within the 90 to 200 pg/ml range when measured in blood. These ranges are general goals. (See chart, page 46.) The HRT prescription that one woman needs in order to maintain these target ranges and to relieve her symptoms may be different from her friend's or her sister's, and the differences could be in *types* of hormones prescribed, *forms* of administration, or in *dosage amounts*.

If a particular medication isn't working, we often hesitate to report it to the doctor, fearing that we'll be thought of as a pest, a bother, or a hypochondriac. Unfortunately, health care providers sometimes seem less than interested in working with us in partnership, which sometimes intimidates us. This was the case with Genevieve, who came to me not long ago to talk over the perimenopausal symptoms she was experiencing and her options for managing them. After we went through her symptoms and family history, she decided that she wanted to try a low dose of HRT that would include natural progesterone and estriol. But when she raised this issue with her health care provider, she heard nothing about the pros and cons of HRT and nothing about taking care of herself. Instead, she was subjected to a lecture during which her physician told her, with practiced condescension, that he "disapproved of doctor shopping."

In Genevieve's situation, one professional's insecurities got in the way of recommending what was best for her. I mention her experience because although many excellent health care providers are willing to take a team approach, some still believe that theirs is the final word. Fortunately, fewer and fewer health care providers adopt a dictatorial style, and fewer patients are willing to accept it when they do. My advice? If you want more than one opinion about your HRT options, give yourself permission to get the information you need. And should you find yourself in a situation like Genevieve's, run—don't walk—out the door.

When Cynthia, a preschool teacher, and her health care provider were attempting to find the best HRT combination for her, she came up with a good analogy for her situation. She had begun on a dosage of 0.25 mg of Estrace twice a day and 200 mg of natural progesterone daily, a combination that relieved her hot flashes and sleeplessness but didn't improve her teary, anxious state of mind. "This reminds me of toddlers," she said. "You think you have everything figured out about their habits and behavior when they're three. Then they turn three and a half, and all bets are off!" The flexibility she adopted in her preschool classes helped her to monitor her symptoms while her HRT was being adjusted and made her unhesitant to let her health care provider know what was going on. Her provider increased her natural progesterone dosage to 300 mg daily, and she found herself in tears much less often.

HOW LONG IS LONG ENOUGH?

"I hate the thought of being on any medication for the rest of my life," said Terri. "I'm only forty-five, and I plan to live until I'm a hundred!" The length of your HRT depends on your history, your symptoms, and your needs. Some women take HRT for a short period of time until specific symptoms, such as hot flashes, are relieved and do not recur. Then they rely on their own sound diet and exercise habits to offset the risks of heart and bone disease. Other women take HRT for years. There is no set number of months or years that works for every woman. The important thing to remember is to take your own "pulse" at least every three months: Are your symptoms being alleviated? How do you feel overall? You can also evaluate the continuation of HRT each time you visit your health care provider: Is it protecting your heart and bones?

What is a reasonable length of time on HRT to provide maximum insurance against heart disease and osteoporosis? HRT will protect your heart and bones only for the time that you take it. Hormones can't be stored in our bodies for later use when we need them — if they could, we wouldn't go through perimenopause or menopause in the first place. Therefore, when HRT is discontinued, its protective action for the heart and bones ends as well. If protecting your heart and bones is a primary concern for you, it may be that you will choose to take HRT for many years but at a low dosage.

NOT CAST IN STONE

Your decision about hormone replacement therapy is a very personal one. Whatever you decide, nothing is cast in stone. If your choice is to try HRT to relieve night sweats, hot flashes, urinary incontinence or mood swings, you can follow up with your health care provider regularly (three months after starting HRT, sooner if any problem occurs). During this follow-up visit, you can evaluate how you are feeling and judge whether your symptoms are adequately relieved. The same holds true if your decision is that HRT is *not* for you right now. At any time, you can always reevaluate, which is why I stress the importance of making a date every three months to check in with yourself and assess how you feel.

One of my patients, Sylvia, found it helpful to take HRT one day at a time. This mentality gave her the open-mindedness she needed to work with her health care provider to decide if she would continue HRT, and to select the best regimen for her.

Obviously, if you feel worse after starting HRT, you don't need to wait for months before you take action. Most women feel the impact of starting, stopping, or adjusting HRT very soon. After starting HRT, symptom relief usually happens within three to four days, and side effects, if they are going to appear, usually show up within three to four days as well. Discontinuing HRT has the same rapid impact: the side effects will go away within a few days, and if HRT has alleviated symptoms such as mood swings or sleeplessness, they often return three to four days after HRT is stopped.

I encounter so many women like Terri who approach the decision about HRT as if it were irrevocable. They fear that they are risking great harm to themselves if they don't make the right decision, or they think that the decision they make today has to stand for the "rest of their lives." I want to emphasize that there is no single "right" decision about HRT, so take that pressure off yourself. What's right for you today may change in the future. The important first steps are to review your history and get all the information you can about HRT. Then talk your options over with a health care provider you trust and who is willing to answer your questions. Most of all, have faith in your own wisdom—the choice you make will be the right one for you.

CHAPTER SEVEN

Complementary Medicine in the Forties

At a certain age, Nature frees women of the child-bearing function, because the rigors of motherhood are more easily borne in earlier years. . . . Instead of being a curb on health and happiness, menopause can leave women freer than she has been since she began menstruating. But for those who do suffer from "hot flashes," irritability and "high strung" feelings, there is a tested way of finding relief.

PACKAGE INSERT FROM A BOTTLE OF LYDIA E. PINKHAM'S VEGETABLE COMPOUND, PATENTED IN 1875 AND MADE IN THE UNITED STATES UNTIL 1968

*L*ydia E. Pinkham's Vegetable Compound, containing a mixture of the herb black cohosh and a prodigious belt of alcohol, is actually a relatively "modern" herbal remedy for menopausal complaints. (The word *perimenopause* had not yet been created.) Only 120 years old, Mrs. Pinkham's tonic for women is a latecomer if we consider the centuries-long span of time that women have used herbs for medicinal and healing purposes. Steeped as tea, crushed, dried, or ground into powder, plants and herbs have been taken or applied by women for hundreds of years in this country, and for thousands of years elsewhere in the world, to ease the pain of childbirth, soothe headaches, alleviate digestive problems, relieve menstrual cramps, improve the skin, eliminate joint pain, induce sleep, and lessen anxiety or depression, to name only a very few uses.

We've seen a recent boom in interest in herbal, "natural," or "alternative" medicine, with best-selling books and major newsmagazine cover stories devoted to the powerful properties of plant-based remedies. In 1992, in a landmark decision, the U.S. government established the Office of Alternative Medicine to provide a formal means of funding research and gathering data on alternatives to conventional medicine.

I prefer the term "complementary" medicine to "alternative"—it eliminates an artificial and unnecessarily adversarial division between so-called conventional or high-tech medicine and other kinds of medicine. I also prefer not to think in terms of "Eastern versus Western medicine" or "big pharmaceutical companies versus ordinary citizens." I don't see an either/or approach, with battle lines drawn between two sides. Rather, I see women in their forties who are resourceful and excited as they research, ask questions, and exchange information about new ways to take charge of their health.

My own interest in complementary approaches started in 1969, when I was part of the childbirth education movement in Milwaukee, Wisconsin. Remember, giving birth without drugs was *very* alternative in those days—some even considered it fringe, or a fad that would soon be over. The "fad" caught on, and what began as a group of seven women became a respected education program that reached hundreds of couples very quickly, an indication of how hungry women were to learn about different ways of giving birth. But this movement wasn't only about having babies—it was about a changed relationship between women and their health care providers.

In my early days as a childbirth education instructor, I got a phone call from a practitioner who wanted me to know that a woman in one of my classes had come into his office with "a list of questions" that he had had to spend "half an hour" answering. "That's great!" I replied enthusiastically, before I realized that he was spluttering with annoyance. The women who made up their minds that they were going to give birth differently from their mothers, or change the experience they had had with the births of their earlier children, really were unstoppable.

It amuses me to recall that some practitioners, when it became clear they couldn't talk any sense into us women, tried to convince our male partners that natural childbirth wasn't a good idea. They would warn a man that if he fainted in the delivery room, they would be forced to attend to him, taking precious time away from his wife and infant. I remember a man in one of my classes who was very alarmed when his wife's practitioner told him to be prepared for "all the screaming and yelling that was going to go on." Women now expect to be offered the option of giving birth without sedation if they choose, and to have the full range of their choices explained to them—it is standard procedure. "Fringe" has been transformed into sound medical practice, all because women decided what they wanted and went about making it happen.

Later in the 1970s I became part of a network of women and health care professionals who introduced the use of natural progesterone into the United States. Unlike synthetic progestins, which were (and still are) widely prescribed, natural progesterone was just beginning to emerge in this country as a treatment with very promising potential for premenstrual syndrome and postpartum depression. The current of energy was very palpable as a handful of us, scattered in different locations in the United States, called and wrote each other (no e-mail or overnight delivery in those days), exchanging information and experiences.

We shared research studies that a group had brought back from England. A select group of patients and doctors were trying natural progesterone, with good early results. It was a tremendously exciting time, because for decades women with premenstrual depression and anxiety had been very harshly judged, labeled neurotic, prescribed tranquilizers, or given a hysterectomy. These were the ones who had summoned the courage to seek help—for every one of them, there were probably ten who silently just thought they were going crazy.

The idea that PMS is a legitimate physiological event in a woman's body was completely foreign to almost all of the medical community when we started exploring options and sharing information. Today we understand much more about cyclical hormone changes and how they affect the way we feel—again, thanks to the determination of a few women and some very caring and intellectually curious professionals.

As I write this book, the women and health care professionals who have shared their views on complementary medicine and perimenopausal health with me can be loosely organized into three groups:

1. Those for whom complementary medicine is a useful first line of offense, an initial step in relieving certain perimenopausal symptoms before exploring prescription options.

2. Those who view complementary medicine as part of a self-care plan, used in conjunction with prescription therapy as a means of additional symptom relief and/or maintenance of well-being.

3. Those for whom hormone replacement therapy is not an option, for personal or medical reasons or both, and who choose complementary medicine as their primary method of care.

I also encounter women who initially explore complementary remedies for perimenopausal symptoms, thinking that it will be easier to buy a product over the counter than to see their health care provider and sort through often contradictory and sometimes alarming information about prescription hormones. But it's not always easier, as Anthea learned.

An engineer who defies every stolid and regimented stereotype of that profession, Anthea has a quick laugh and a sharp wit that sometimes goes right past people. "I heard an ad," she told me, "on my car radio for a vitamin or herb, I'm not sure which, that supposedly gives you your life back, or something like that. The woman in the ad sounds whiny and nasal at first, but by the end of the ad she sounds throaty and sexy as she's telling you how midlife is now miraculous, thanks to this product."

"Madison Avenue should love me," Anthea continued, "because there I was, driving right to the health food store to see if I could find this stuff." Once inside, Anthea found not only the product she had heard about on the radio but several others like it, many with similar ingredients. "I couldn't tell exactly what the difference was between them," she said. "The young woman working there was very earnest and helpful, and she showed me at least a dozen other creams, vitamins, tinctures, and herbs. I realized I didn't know enough about what I was looking for and decided to come back after I had done some reading."

A few weeks earlier, Anthea had celebrated her forty-seventh birthday. The radio ad for the midlife miracle had lured her because she could no longer ignore nightly restlessness and hot flashes during the day. When she came to see me, her annual physical showed that she was in excellent health, but her symptoms suggested that her hormone levels were changing. "I'm interested in seeing if a vitamin or herb might be enough to control these symptoms until my body adjusts," she said.

There is a wealth of complementary options for managing perimenopause symptoms. One challenge for Anthea would come in deciding:

- what to take
- how much to take, and in what combination with other medications
- when to take it
- if there are side effects
- where to find a quality product

We'll review some of the complementary approaches to perimenopausal health that are generating lots of interest and excitement among women and their health care providers today. We'll look at what research has been done in certain areas, and where the potential for future investigation lies. We'll also talk about working with your health care provider in selecting and trying complementary remedies.

WHY DON'T I KNOW ABOUT THIS?

When I first mentioned Remifemin (a formulation of black cohosh) to my patient Janice as a possibility for managing her insomnia and hot flashes, she wanted to know why she hadn't heard of it. "Is it new?"

"No, black cohosh has been used for centuries by Native Americans, usually for menstrual cramps. Remifemin has been used in Germany for more than forty years. It's less widely used in this country — the majority of health care providers still aren't familiar with it."

"Do I need a prescription for it?"

I explained to Janice that her health care provider could prescribe Remifemin, but that it's also available as an over-the-counter product. The Food and Drug Administration (FDA) considers Remifemin a food supplement rather than a medication, which means that it's not subject to the approval process that a synthesized medication has to go through before it can be marketed. But the FDA also prohibits suppliers of "food supplements," including Remifemin, from making medical claims on the label. Thus the FDA doesn't tell us if an herb or vitamin like Remifemin is safe or effective.

In Germany, on the other hand, a government commission (Commission E) plays a stricter watchdog role, reviewing clinical data about herbal remedies, verifying claims made by manufacturers, and issuing statements on the safety and effectiveness of more than three hundred herbs. (No government agency plays this role in the United States, but the German Commission E report will soon be translated and available here for the first time.)

The FDA approval process is lengthy and expensive. A drug manufacturer must submit data to the FDA, and these data must meet stringent requirements. The process usually takes many years, and its estimated costs range from $100 million to $450 million. Most drug manufacturers recoup these staggering research and development costs with profits from drug sales, and there's the rub: herbal remedies can't be patented. Even if a manufacturer of an herbal remedy could come up with $100 million to pay for the research and testing necessary for the FDA approval process, it would have no way to offset these costs through exclusive sales of the herbal product. The market is wide open for anyone to copy and sell herbal remedies. Thus, even if the FDA decided to begin overseeing herb, vitamin, and mineral safety, manufacturers would have little incentive to go through the approval process.

The approval process is only part of the reason why some of us are less familiar with plant-based remedies. Many health care providers' training includes little or no information about the use of plants and herbs as healing substances, except those providers who were trained as naturopathic or homeopathic doctors. But there is growing interest in, and acceptance of, the use of herbs and plants, and more and more women are choosing to consult herbalists to help them select the appropriate preparations.

PARTNERSHIPS IN HEALTH

Among the women I talk to, there's a buzz of excitement and lots of networking as we look for ways to make our perimenopausal transition very different from our mothers'. Never mind that relieving perimenopausal symptoms with herbs still isn't standard practice — we've taken the initiative, done lots of research on our own, experimented with what works, and shared the information with friends, sisters, co-workers, and neighbors.

Evaluating complementary remedies requires the same kind of vigilance we use when we evaluate any prescription hormone option for perimenopause. As I have done my own investigation about herbal remedies, talked with professionals and women who use them, and tried them myself, these principles have been helpful in choosing among the many, many, complementary products available to us now:

+ Decide which symptoms you most want to manage. That will help you prioritize among certain products.

+ Educate yourself about including herbal or complementary remedies in your self-care plan. Start by doing some reading on your own. (*The Healing Power of Herbs* by Michael T. Murray, N.D., *Herbs of Choice* by Varro E. Tyler, and *The Lawrence Review of Natural Products*, a newsletter, are excellent resources.)

+ Enlist the help of a knowledgeable professional who can guide you as you select, combine, and monitor the effects of the herbs you choose. You may have to do some searching to find an individual who has a thorough background in herbal or plant-based remedies (see appendix B).

+ Keep in mind that *herbal* is not a synonym for *benign*, and that in fact some plants are highly toxic, even deadly. Never assume that a herbal or natural preparation is harmless; thoroughly investigate everything you are going to put in your body.

+ Bring your health care provider into the loop. While more and more people are exploring complementary or alternative approaches to a host of health issues, research shows that two-thirds of them do not inform their primary health care provider about their explorations. I strongly recommend that you include your provider in your search, for two important reasons. First, he or she can help you determine if any medication you are taking would interact adversely with an herbal preparation. (Herbs can interact with each other and other medicines, specifically antidepressants, anti-anxiety agents, and some medications to control high blood pressure, to name a few.) Second, your experiences may help your provider learn about and become more receptive to nondrug approaches.

- ✦ If you are pregnant or are trying to become pregnant, be very cautious about taking natural preparations, just as you would be with any medication. Unless you and your health care provider can be 100 percent certain that a medication or herb will have absolutely no effect on your fetus, my suggestion is not to take it while you are trying to conceive or during your pregnancy.

- ✦ Read labels carefully. The quality of some herbal preparations varies widely. If the label makes it hard to understand how much of a particular herb or other ingredient is in a product, look for another brand.

- ✦ Remember that some herbs or plant-based medicines exert very potent influences on the body. (The heart medication digitalis, for example, is derived from plants in the nightshade family.) Be sure you understand how much of the herb you need to take, and never assume that "more is better."

- ✦ Be a wise consumer. Just as no prescription hormone will be a cure-all or silver bullet for all perimenopausal symptoms, the same is true for herbs and other complementary medicines. If a claim seems exaggerated, it probably is. Also, you need to look at any herbal remedy as part of a larger picture that includes your lifestyle.

- ✦ Quality control isn't always easy with herbal products. In my experience, I have found that PhytoPharmica in Green Bay, Wisconsin, and Celestial Seasonings in Boulder, Colorado, are both reliable sources that rigorously test their products to ensure quality.

- ✦ I also recommend comparing costs. Good health can never be too expensive, of course, but before you buy any product or preparation that has a high cost, be sure you have solid evidence that it is going to do what you expect.

- ✦ Finally, when you decide to try a new approach, think about timing. I generally advise against trying something brand new when the stakes are very high — like trying a remedy for insomnia the night before a big presentation or other important event when you're very concerned about getting rest. If you don't get the desired result right away, your disappointment stands to be much greater.

PHYTOESTROGENS IN PERIMENOPAUSE

In looking at the specific herbs that can be beneficial in managing peri-menopausal symptoms, I want to begin with an explanation of phyto-estrogens. A phytoestrogen (*phyto* means "plant") is a plant or herb that can exert estrogenlike effects in the body. Its activity is relatively weak compared with that of estrogen taken as a medication. (Prescription estrogen is a hundred times stronger than phytoestrogens.)

Phytoestrogens can almost be described as having a brain, since these plants and herbs appear both to exert and to balance estrogenic effects. For example, if estrogen levels are low, phytoestrogens seem to exert an estrogenic effect. If estrogen levels are high, phytoestrogens appear to occupy estrogen receptor sites in the body, "fooling" the body into believing it has enough estrogen and exerting a braking mechanism on the production of more. Phytoestrogens are used to help regulate both physical and emotional symptoms of perimenopause. I'll discuss herbs for the most part in this chapter, and phytoestrogenic foods in chapter 8.

MOOD SWINGS AND HERBS

I see many women in my practice in whom the physical symptoms of perimenopause, such as headaches, vaginal dryness, and hot flashes, are either absent or cause minimal interruption in their lives, but who find themselves unpleasantly buffeted by changing moods. If such a woman is interested in trying an herbal preparation to help balance her moods, I always start by reviewing what she is eating and when, and how much exercise she is able to incorporate into her day. Unfortunately, no herb can undo the effects of a diet that's lacking in essential nutrients or make up for a sedentary lifestyle. After we complete this review, we go on to discuss herbs if she chooses.

ANXIETY

I have had Nina as a patient for ten years; I first saw her when she was in her midthirties, when she came to me for help with premenstrual syndrome. At that time we devised a program for her then that included, along with balancing her diet and increasing her exercise, the occasional use of natural progesterone. I hadn't seen her in more than a year when she came in again recently. She looked very troubled as she said, "I don't know what's going on. My PMS has gotten really bad—even worse than it was ten years ago. I'm so anxious, I literally feel like I'm jumping out of my skin. Nothing is working anymore."

Nina is 44 now, and the grade-school children she had when she first came to my office are in college. She and I talked about how fluctuating hormone levels in the forties can manifest themselves as worsening PMS, particularly if a woman still has a regular cycle.

When Nina said "nothing is working," she meant that she was avoiding sweets, alcohol, salt, and caffeine as much as possible and still maintaining a regular exercise routine. (She and her husband spend many weekends mountain biking, and she rides during the week.) Yet in spite of her efforts, she said, "I get this terrible feeling in the pit of my stomach. Sometimes I almost feel like I'm going to get sick. I've tried deep breathing, but I can't seem to calm down."

Nina shook her head when I asked if there were any unusual stresses or pressures in her life. "Not really. Nothing that hasn't been there before. Money is really tight with two kids in college, but we're managing."

Since Nina's primary goal was to get a handle on her anxiety, I suggested that she might want to try black cohosh to bring her moods more into balance. Black cohosh is used for a variety of symptoms during perimenopause, including hot flashes and insomnia, but it has also been shown to be useful in relieving anxiety. Nina had the option of taking black cohosh in several forms, either as a tea, as a fluid or powdered extract, or as a standardized product, Remifemin, which my patient Janice is also taking. Black cohosh is believed to suppress luteinizing hormone levels in the body, which may spike irregularly as estrogen levels fall.

I am comfortable recommending Remifemin to my patients who are interested in using black cohosh for several reasons. First, it is a standardized formula that has been studied for four decades in Germany.

Second, it has been shown to help alleviate a variety of menopausal symptoms, and some women prefer to take one preparation for broad symptom relief rather than individual herbs or vitamins targeted at specific symptoms. Also, with Remifemin it is easier for patients to monitor exactly how much black cohosh they are taking. I suggested that Nina begin with a dose of 40 mg per day and keep a chart of her symptoms to evaluate its effect on her symptoms for one month.

It usually takes about two weeks to begin to experience relief from perimenopausal symptoms with Remifemin. Dosage amounts range from 40 to 80 mg per day. I generally suggest that women begin at the low end of the dosage range and increase the amount if their symptoms are not relieved within two weeks. I do not recommend taking above 80 mg per day. When I saw Nina one month later she said 40 mg daily seemed to be adequate for her. She was experiencing less anxiety.

Ilse also found that black cohosh was very helpful in controlling palpitations that made her feel as if she were having a panic attack or, worse, a heart attack. A successful real estate saleswoman, Ilse almost left her job because she was having increasing episodes where her heart would race without warning. "I had appointment after appointment with this specialist and that specialist," she told me. "I didn't have heart disease, they told me. Someone finally called it anxiety disorder or something like that. I still have a prescription for an anti-anxiety medication, but I put it in my drawer and never filled it. It's not that I didn't want to take it, but I had this gut feeling that something else was going on besides anxiety."

She found out about black cohosh from a friend of hers and tried it on her own. After using 160 mg daily (two 40 mg tablets morning and evening) for six months, she said that "black cohosh took care of the palpitations almost a hundred percent. I felt much better after using it for only two weeks."

When Ilse told her health care provider she was using black cohosh, "I got a funny look from her. But she has to admit that I'm doing much better. For a while I was in and out of her office all the time because I didn't know what was going on, and neither did she."

Black cohosh was Ilse's choice as a first line of treatment for peri-menopausal heart palpitations. Other women start taking HRT, then decide they would like to switch to black cohosh to see if it will take care of their symptoms. The transition from HRT to black cohosh should be made gradually over a five-to-eight-week period, following these steps:

1. Evaluate the importance of heart and bone protection with your health care provider. Black cohosh probably does not provide this protection. If your cardiovascular health is not an issue but your goal is to build bone strength, black cohosh can be taken with natural progesterone, which has bone-building properties.

2. Begin adding soy to your diet (see chapter 8), and be certain you are getting adequate amounts of calcium daily (1500 mg). Boosting your soy and calcium intake is a gentle and natural way to protect your heart and bones.

3. Begin taking black cohosh (40 mg daily to begin) while you are still taking HRT.

4. For the first three to four weeks of the combined HRT/black cohosh regimen, gradually taper your dosage of estrogen. For instance, if you have been taking 1 mg of estrogen daily, take 1 mg one day and 0.5 mg every other day. Remember that you must continue to take a form of progesterone even as you taper down your estrogen, and that you are still taking black cohosh daily. Continue to take progesterone at your regular dosage; do not taper down the dosage of this hormone.

5. After three to four weeks, reduce your estrogen again, taking half your normal dosage every day. Follow this reduced estrogen dosage for two to three weeks, continuing with the black cohosh.

6. Then for one week, take half of your normal dosage of estrogen every other day. You may then discontinue the estrogen and take black cohosh along with progesterone if you choose. Black cohosh does not have to be opposed by progesterone the way

estrogen does, but some women choose to take the combination of black cohosh with progesterone.

The literature on black cohosh states that its side effects are minimal—a very few patients will report stomach upset. But I have heard a few women report that the maximum dosage of 160 mg per day made them feel like their breasts were engorged. If this occurs, lowering the dose to 80 mg per day should take care of the side effect. Although no toxic effects are associated with black cohosh, you may want to use it to provide short-term relief from specific symptoms.

MORE SOURCES OF CALM

Other preparations to ease anxiety include valerian and kava. The root of the perennial plant valerian is the portion that is used medicinally to produce a calming effect and to treat anxiety. Valerian's sedative effect is believed to be due to the presence of valeric acid in the root. Experts recommend using a water-soluble valerian extract, standardized to contain 0.8 percent valeric acid. Valerian root has a very strong unpleasant smell, but odor-free preparations are available. A daily dosage of 150 to 300 mg of valerian extract acts as a mild sedative for some people, although I have spoken with women who found valerian too potent for them. "It knocked me out," said Michelle.

There is also some evidence that valerian can have a stimulatory effect—it has been used to counteract extreme fatigue. One expert I consulted said that valerian's effects depend on the way it is prepared. When the root is dried, it can have stimulatory rather than calming effects. If you decide to try valerian to relieve anxiety, you'll want to be sure to choose a preparation that will have calming, not stimulating effects.

Also used to produce a calming effect, kava is a member of the pepper family that grows widely on many Pacific islands. Traditional rituals and ceremonies on many of these islands include sharing a drink made from root of kava. The active ingredient in kava is the kava lactones, which appear to act on the central nervous system. Some women choose to try kava instead of prescription anti-anxiety medications such as the benzodiazepines Valium or Xanax.

An extract containing 70 percent kava lactones may be taken three times daily (dosages range from 45 to 70 mg) or before bedtime (180 to 210 mg). Overconsumption of kava results in a condition called kava dermopathy (scaly dry skin). As with any herbal preparation, more than the recommended amount of kava should not be taken. Kava is also contraindicated in people who have Parkinson's disease.

DEPRESSION

Karen is the midforties woman with the solid marriage, children she adores, and stable home life whose persistent feelings of depression both bewildered her and made her feel guilty, as if she should snap out of it. As I had recommended, Karen had a thorough physical exam. Her overall health was very good, and her hormone levels were just slightly below normal ranges—not low enough for her to want to take replacement hormones now. She also hesitated to take the antidepressant medication that her health care provider suggested.

"This may seem silly or like I'm in denial, but somehow I have this feeling that taking antidepressants is for people who are really much worse off than I am. I'd rather wait and see if these feelings will pass on their own, or take something less intimidating than antidepressants."

Karen's sister had given her a book on the herb St. John's wort, which is reported to be very effective in treating mild to moderate depression. Like black cohosh, St. John's wort has been well researched and is widely prescribed in Germany. Karen found the idea that an herb might help lift her depression appealing, and she called her health care provider to ask about it: "There was a little beat of silence on the other end of the phone. But when I said I'd like to try it for a couple of months to see if it made a difference, he said he respected my choice and didn't see any harm in it. Actually I think he might be curious too."

The active ingredient in St. John's wort, a perennial plant, is hypericin. It was originally believed that St. John's wort inhibited a type of brain enzyme called monoamine oxidase (MAO). Dampening MAO levels is the principle behind a very powerful group of drugs called MAO inhibitors. But as more research on St. John's wort has been done in Europe, it appears now that this herb may inhibit serotonin reuptake.

You'll remember that serotonin is the brain chemical with a significant influence on mood. When reuptake of serotonin is inhibited, the chemical's "feel good" effects in the brain last longer. Drugs such as Prozac, Zoloft, and Paxil belong to the class of medications known as selective serotonin reuptake inhibitors, or SSRIs.

Karen started taking a standard extract of St. John's wort (0.3 percent hypericin), beginning with the standard dosage of 300 mg three times daily. She took it with meals to minimize the possibility of gastric upset. "I feel good," she said with enthusiasm when I called to see how she was doing a month later. "For one thing, I'm glad I had a physical so I can be assured nothing is wrong with me. It also gave me more of a sense of control to decide to try St. John's wort first before I go on to anything else. Maybe I won't need anything else, because I really do feel like there's less of a cloud hanging over me. When I felt that way, there was usually nothing I could really put my finger on, but I just knew I wasn't myself."

Karen said she wouldn't call St. John's wort a miracle, but one measure of how it was working for her after only four weeks might be that her husband and one of her children noticed a change: "My husband said, 'You seem more like yourself.' I also heard my oldest daughter tell one of her friends on the phone that yes, maybe I would drive them somewhere, because I've been in a better mood lately." She gave a slight laugh. "I guess the ultimate barometer of how I'm doing is my teenager's assessment of my mood," she said drily.

Because Karen has olive skin and very dark hair and eyes, she doesn't have to be cautious about sensitivity to sunlight, which St. John's wort causes in animals that graze on the plant. But even though photosensitivity has not been reported in humans, fair-skinned individuals with light skin and eyes are advised to avoid strong sunlight and other ultraviolet light when they are taking St. John's wort.

While much of the attention focused on St. John's wort examines its use to alleviate depression, this herb may be useful in reducing anxiety as well. As more is understood about the effect of St. John's wort on serotonin levels and mood, we stand to see substantial increase in its application and use in this country. But I am somewhat concerned about branding St. John's wort as the alternative to Prozac for two reasons. First, we don't yet know that St. John's wort will be effective in helping severely depressed people — it appears most effective in people with mild to moderate depression. Second, I am no more comfortable with widespread, cavalier, uninformed use of an herbal preparation than I am with such use of a prescription medication, so I worry about the idea that we can all take an herb, or a pill of any kind for that matter, and expect it to put our lives in order.

I've mentioned black cohosh for use in connection with hot flashes and anxiety, among other perimenopausal symptoms. But the German research shows that this herb also reduces feelings of depression in perimenopausal women. When using black cohosh for depression, the dosage is two 40 mg tablets per day.

Sleep Disturbances

Black cohosh can also help produce more restful sleep, although researchers haven't yet isolated the exact mechanism by which it does so. We know that it evens out the production of luteinizing hormone, which works hand in hand with FSH, the hormone implicated in hot flashes and night sweats. Fewer night sweats may be the reason some women sleep better when they are taking black cohosh; for others, the herb's ability to reduce anxiety and depression means fewer nights lying awake feeling worried or morose.

Janice is using a standardized preparation of black cohosh to help control her hot flashes, but it may also be helping her to sleep better, along with her calcium citrate supplement, which she now takes in the evening. Two months after she started keeping a record of how she was feeling, I reviewed her symptom chart with her, and the change in her sleep patterns was evident. The notations of "insomnia" were much less frequent.

The anti-anxiety herbs valerian and kava are also said to help people sleep more easily and restfully (see "Depression," above). Passion flower is also widely used in Europe as a mild sedative or to help induce sleep, although this remedy is less studied than St. John's wort and black cohosh. Dried passion flower is usually taken as a tea (4 to 8 g per serving).

Another calming tea that I often use to help wind down and pre-pare for sleep is made from chamomile. I value the ritual as much as the properties of the chamomile itself: taking time to sit quietly by myself, sip tea from my favorite mug, which one of my sons made for me years ago in a grade-school ceramics class, and let go of the day's cares.

Not an herb, melatonin is often used to promote sleep, and some consider it an alternative or complementary approach to sleep distur-bances. As I mentioned in chapter 4, melatonin is a hormone produced by the pineal gland. It can be useful for the short-term treatment of jet lag (3 to 5 mg taken in the destination time zone), but I suggest caution about taking it daily. Over-the-counter melatonin products often con-tain very high levels of this hormone, much more than your body would produce naturally.

In fact, whether it's melatonin, an herb, or a prescription sedative, my approach toward sleep aids is to view them as short-term or occa-sional measures rather than something to rely on all the time. Ideally, you should not have to take any preparation on a regular basis in order to sleep. Breaking the cycle of insomnia can often be accomplished with short-term use (one week or less) of an herb; then your body's natural sleep rhythm is restored. (See chapter 4 for other hints on sleeping well during perimenopause.)

FORGETFULNESS AND TROUBLE CONCENTRATING

For some women, perimenopausal forgetfulness or changes in their abil-ity to concentrate are extremely troubling, especially when we don't connect these changes to hormonal fluctuations. Sometimes these symptoms of impaired concentration come at the same time we are observing age-related changes in our elderly parents, and we can won-der if we are prematurely losing our edge or suddenly becoming less sharp. Many women have confided in me that they were worried they were developing Alzheimer's disease.

When Janice found herself sometimes going over and over the numbers that she was responsible for crunching at her firm, losing track of where she was and having to start over again in preparing the complicated reports that she regularly produced as part of her job, she decided to try ginkgo biloba to improve her mental concentration. She also took black cohosh to help with perimenopausal hot flashes.

The leaves of this ancient decorative tree, ginkgo biloba, have a rich history of medicinal use. In China ginkgo leaves have been used for literally thousands of years to increase blood flow to the brain. Today ginkgo biloba leaf extracts are very commonly prescribed in Germany and France.

What we know about ginkgo's workings in the body is largely based on animal research. Clinical trials with humans have examined ginkgo's effects on a variety of symptoms and conditions, including memory loss, depression, macular degeneration (a cause of blindness in adults), certain hearing problems, and tinnitus (ringing of the ears), among others.

In animals, it has been shown that ginkgo biloba extract affects the lining of the blood vessels, and in humans, researchers believe it improves cerebral blood flow. In a very simplified summary, it could be said that by boosting the flow of blood and oxygen to the brain, ginkgo stimulates and improves certain brain functions, some of which are related to our ability to recall certain facts.

In his book *The Healing Power of Herbs,* naturopathic doctor Michael T. Murray states that clinical research indicates that ginkgo should be taken consistently for at least twelve weeks to be effective. After taking 120 mg of ginkgo daily (three 40 mg capsules), for eight weeks, Janice said she felt some improvement in her ability to concentrate: "Let's just say I haven't hit the wall at three o'clock recently. For a while, by late afternoon, I would be in my office with the door closed, taking twice as long as usual to do one small task and sometimes sitting there for a good two or three minutes trying to remember what I was supposed to do next."

Janice acknowledged that along with taking ginkgo, she had also made a serious effort in the previous month to reorganize and reprioritize her workload, delegating certain responsibilities and asking her assistant to step up her share of the duties. "It's been great for both of us," she told me. "I've realized that I don't have to do everything, and she seems to appreciate the trust I have in her."

It's not clear which helped Janice's ability to concentrate more: ginkgo or reordering some of her work. She did point out, however, that reorganizing her workload and providing explicit instructions to her assistant "took a lot of clear thinking." Looking at me over the top of her glasses, Janice said, "Maybe the ginkgo helped me think all that through. Once I had a picture in my mind of how I wanted things done, I had to be able to write some of it down and explain the rest articulately. I'm not sure I could have done that two or three months ago, I felt so muddled at times."

If you try ginkgo, look for an extract that contains 24 percent ginkgo flavone glycosides. Few side effects are associated with ginkgo, and these occur only infrequently (gastric upset, headache, and dizziness). One of my patients did report headaches when she took ginkgo, but she switched to a different brand and took it without any side effect.

In relation to improving memory and concentration, I also want to talk briefly about DHEA (dehydroepiandrosterone). Like melatonin, DHEA is not an herb but a hormone, and it is widely available as an over-the-counter preparation. It is called a precursor or foundation hormone because in the body it "cascades" or turns into other hormones, including testosterone and estrogen. In adults, DHEA levels begin dropping at about age twenty. Some researchers believe that restoring DHEA to youthful levels can delay the effects of aging, notably memory loss and impaired concentration. Some scientific data also found that DHEA lowered the death rate from cardiovascular disease in men (results that have not yet been repeated in women).

DHEA is sometimes discussed as a preparation that can minimize several perimenopausal symptoms in addition to memory loss: bone loss, fatigue, vaginal dryness, sleeplessness, and dry skin. Using DHEA for perimenopausal symptoms is sometimes based on the theory that this precursor hormone will cascade into estrogen and thus alleviate symptoms produced by estrogen deficiency. It's not that simple, however. First of all, not all scientists agree that taking DHEA as a supplement will produce the same cascade effects. Assuming that DHEA supplements will cascade into other hormones also assumes that all the other chemicals and enzymes needed are present in the body, and we can't know this.

If you're thinking about trying DHEA, I have two recommendations:

- Have your DHEA levels measured first in blood or saliva to determine how much of the hormone your body is currently producing. As is true with any hormone, you wouldn't want to take more if your body is still producing a normal level.
- Work with a health care professional who is knowledgeable about DHEA supplementation so you can arrive at the dosage appropriate for you. Recommended DHEA dosages for women range from 5 to 50 mg daily.

HERBS FOR HOT FLASHES

"I've had night sweats for a year at least, now that I think back," said Heidi. "They got to the point where they were really annoying, waking me up in the middle of the night several times a week." Night sweats are hot flashes that happen at night—flushing, feeling very hot, and perspiring. Some women have palpitations or feel dizzy and shaky during a hot flash.

Hot flashes are harder to overlook or dismiss than some other perimenopausal symptoms. While we may attribute certain symptoms to fatigue or stress, we can't really avoid confronting a soaked nightgown or blouse in the aftermath of a night sweat or hot flash. For Heidi, night sweats were the signal that she was perimenopausal, although until she came to see me, she thought hot flashes meant menopause.

Heidi is a children's librarian, and she has a way of relating incidents in her life to stories and fables she loves. "There's a wonderful girls' book where three friends talk about getting their periods. One of them is very reluctant to mature, and she screams, 'If anyone thinks I'm gonna do anything like that, they're crazy.'"

When Heidi realized that her night sweats weren't getting any better, the word *menopause* seemed to blink like a neon sign in front of her: "I thought of Harriet—if anyone thinks I'm going to do menopause at forty-six, they're crazy."

Heidi wanted to try a combination of the herbs angelica, chaste berry, licorice, and black cohosh to see if it would help her night sweats. But black cohosh alone can work well to minimize hot flashes and night sweats — Janice, for one, found it to be very effective. Surges of heat during the day had been causing Janice to perspire through her clothes frequently, making her a favored customer as she marched into the dry cleaner regularly with armloads of jackets and blouses. She started taking 80 mg of black cohosh daily. Janice liked to do things by the numbers, and when I asked her after two months if her hot flashes had improved, she replied, "I balanced my checkbook a few days ago. I'm writing half the number of checks to my dry cleaner that I was last year at this time." She has seen a very noticeable reduction in hot flashes.

Black cohosh can also be combined with other herbs to curb hot flashes, as Heidi wanted. Several preparations containing two or more herbs are marketed as helpful in relieving symptoms of perimenopause or menopause. Along with black cohosh they may include:

+ Angelica. The Chinese version of angelica, dong quai, is often used to minimize hot flashes. Both Chinese and Japanese angelicas are phytoestrogens, and they may work to reduce hot flashes by exerting some estrogenic activity in the body. When used alone, angelica is taken three times daily as a powder or tea (1 to 2 g), a tincture (1 tsp.) or a fluid extract (¼ tsp.).

+ Chaste tree berry. This herb, as the name suggests, was given to women in ancient times to dampen their libido. Research on chaste tree berry is limited — there is some suggestion that an extract of it lowers production of the hormone prolactin. The recommended chaste tree berry dosage is 20 mg per day.

+ Licorice. The root of this perennial also has a centuries-long history of medicinal use. The active ingredient in licorice root is glycyrrhizin. Like soy, licorice contains isoflavones, substances that have the dual effect of exerting an estrogenic effect if estrogen levels are low, or inhibiting estrogen action if estrogen levels are high. Among its many uses, licorice is sometimes used to relieve PMS or menstrual cramps. There are no research studies with humans documenting that licorice will help hot flashes, but some women report that licorice, taken alone or in combination with other herbs, provides relief from this perimenopausal symptom.

Taken for too long or in doses that are too high, licorice can have very serious side effects, including hypertension. This herb should not be used by individuals who have high blood pressure, cardiovascular disease, or kidney disease, and in general it should not be used for more than one month. Usually taken three times a day, licorice dosages are as follows: powdered root (1 to 2 g), fluid extract (2 to 4 ml), dry extract (250 to 500 mg). To avoid side effects or interaction with other medications, be sure to monitor the use of licorice carefully with help from a knowledgeable professional. If you choose, you can select a product that combines recommended amounts of licorice, angelica, chaste tree berry, and black cohosh. That's what Heidi did, and she did see improvement in her hot flashes and night sweats. They didn't stop altogether, but she said they were less frequent.

+ Oil of evening primrose. Known more for its role in relieving PMS, evening primrose oil is also sometimes used to relieve hot flashes. It contains gamma linolenic acid, which is a precursor of hormonelike substances called prostaglandins. Like cholesterol, there are "good" and "bad" types of prostaglandins, and evening primrose oil raises blood levels of PGE1, the "good" prostaglandin. PGE1 mediates the effect of the "bad" prostaglandin, PGE2, which is linked to painful menstrual cramps. Recommended dosages of evening primrose oil range from 500 to 2000 mg per day. The Efamol brand has a good reputation among women who use evening primrose oil, but it is expensive.

GENITOURINARY SYMPTOMS

As estrogen's nourishing effects decline, vaginal tissue can become thin and dry, more subject to unfriendly bacteria and infection. Vaginal stinging or burning can be very uncomfortable, and intercourse can become unpleasant or even painful. Vitamin E, taken orally or applied as an oil directly to the vagina, is a natural remedy that some women choose for vaginal dryness.

The herbs uva ursi and goldenseal are also sometimes used to treat urinary tract infections. Uva ursi's most active ingredient, arbutin, acts as an antibiotic in the urinary tract when taken three times daily as a tea (1.5 to 4 g), tincture (4 to 6 ml), fluid extract (0.5 to 2.0 ml), or solid extract (250 to 500 mg). Uva ursi can be toxic if taken in excess, inducing nausea, shortness of breath, and in extreme cases, loss of consciousness. The dried root of the goldenseal plant is sometimes used in combination with uva ursi to alleviate pain or burning upon urination. The active ingredient in goldenseal is berberine.

HORMONAL HEADACHES

As I mentioned earlier, headache experts believe that perimenopausal headaches are linked less to changes in the amounts of hormones present in our bodies than to abrupt shifts and fluctuations in the levels of estrogen and progesterone. This perimenopausal symptom can be tricky to manage, and many women have tried several medications without success. Hormone replacement therapy clears up hormonally related headaches in many women, but for those who would choose a complementary remedy instead, the herb feverfew shows some promise as a remedy to prevent and treat migraine.

Feverfew is a member of the sunflower family. In two British clinical trials, capsules containing dried feverfew leaves were more effective than placebo. An important note about feverfew: the active ingredient is parthenolide. A daily dosage to prevent migraine must contain at least 0.25 to 0.5 mg of this ingredient. Many products that are available over the counter and are marketed as herbal headache remedies contain little or none of this essential ingredient.

CHANGES IN SEX DRIVE

There's something fun about the idea of using an aphrodisiac to stimulate sex drive, although many of the women who come to Full Circle

Women's Health for help with perimenopausal changes in sex drive are also struggling with depression or fatigue and are not exactly having fun with much of anything.

I don't generally recommend an herbal approach as a first line of offense against a waning sex drive. In my experience, lack of libido in the forties is usually complex, intertwined with hormonal shifts and life issues as well. In this complicated and deeply personal area, I prefer to start with a broader approach than treating the symptom by itself. However, I certainly do not oppose it if a woman is set on trying an herb first.

These herbal preparations are believed to be helpful in stimulating sex drive:

+ Damiana, also known as old woman's broom. The Aztec Indians are reported to have used damiana as an aphrodisiac. It can be drunk as a tea and is also found in combination herbal preparations.

+ False unicorn root. Long used as a remedy for menstrual problems, false unicorn root is said to have aphrodisiac qualities, although there are no data to substantiate this claim. It was an ingredient in Mrs. Pinkham's Vegetable Compound.

+ Siberian ginseng. This herb is often recommended as a general tonic, and the Chinese believe that its regular use is good for overall health. But there are no studies associating Siberian ginseng with increased libido. It may be that women who find it helpful in increasing their overall energy and well-being also experience the ripple effect of restarting a stalled sex drive. Note that there are many types of ginseng—Siberian ginseng is just one of several varieties. Their quality varies widely. A Siberian ginseng extract of 33 percent ethanol can be taken three times daily as a dry extract (100 to 200 mg), fluid extract (2.0 to 4.0 ml), a dried root (2 to 4 g), or a tincture (10 to 20 ml). This herb is usually taken for 60 days or less, with a two-to-three-week interval before starting the herb again. Avoid taking more than the recommended amounts of ginseng, as side effects can occur, including mood swings, sleeplessness, and depression.

Other Complementary Treatments for Perimenopausal Symptoms

ACUPUNCTURE

The practice of acupuncture is based on the Chinese philosophy that physical and emotional problems result from an imbalance or interruption in the flow of *chi,* or life energy, through the body. Chi is said to flow through meridians or channels, and very specific points along these meridians are associated with symptoms and emotions. In acupuncture, ultrafine needles are inserted painlessly into points on the body that correspond with the symptom or problem a person reports. Some women find acupuncture helpful in treating migraines, hot flashes, or changes in menstrual flow associated with perimenopausal hormone shifts. Chinese herbal remedies are sometimes used in combination with acupuncture.

The regulation and licensing of acupuncture practitioners varies from state to state. If you are interested in acupuncture, you can start by contacting your local department of health to find out about this practice in your state. When you find a practitioner of acupuncture and/or Chinese herbal medicine, you'll want to inquire about background, training, and certification. You may also want to ask for references, so you can speak to another perimenopausal woman treated by this practitioner.

HOMEOPATHIC REMEDIES

The subject of homeopathy is a hard one for me. I have seen women in my practice who are also under the care of a homeopathic health care provider and who believe very strongly that homeopathy is beneficial for them. I encounter equal numbers of women and health care providers who are very dubious about its value. I don't think there is one simple black-and-white way to look at homeopathy. When I do see a woman who is either already pursuing homeopathic options or wants to do so, I keep an open mind, try to learn what I can, and direct her to the appropriate resources in her community.

If this is an avenue you are interested in exploring, I would advise you to seek help from a reliable professional who has experience in working with homeopathic remedies for perimenopausal symptoms (see appendix B). It is not my goal here either to advocate or preach against homeopathy; instead I will briefly explain how it is said to work and provide a very basic overview of some common ingredients in homeopathic remedies used for perimenopausal symptoms.

Homeopathy is built on the idea that the body's natural healing process produces symptoms that should not be repressed. In the early 1800s, the founding father of homeopathy, the German physician Samuel Hahnemann, discovered that quinine, which was used to treat malaria, also produced malaria symptoms. Hahnemann began experimenting with the concept that tiny amounts of certain natural substances could have curative effects.

Homeopathic preparations are made using a process called *succussion*, or vigorous shaking. For example, suppose a "10X" preparation of sepia is to be made. Sepia, a pigment obtained from the secretion of the cuttlefish, is said to be helpful in alleviating vaginal dryness. One drop of sepia is added to 10 drops of distilled water and shaken vigorously. One drop of this solution is then added to another ten drops of water. The process is repeated a total of ten times, each time with the succussion, to create a "10X" sepia preparation.

Critics of homeopathy argue that, by the laws of physics, no therapeutic amount of any substance could remain in such a dilute preparation. Those schooled in homeopathy contend that the process of shaking releases energy from the original substance and transmits this energy into the molecules of the distilled water. The release of this energy provides a solution's healing power, according to homeopathic experts.

Hundreds of homeopathic remedies combine certain substances for particular conditions, and perimenopause is among them, although most of these combination preparations say they are for "menopause." Black cohosh (usually identified as *cimicifuga racemosaex* in homeopathic preparations) is sometimes taken by perimenopausal women in very small homeopathic amounts. Some other common ingredients of homeopathic remedies for women with hormonally related symptoms are listed here, although this list is by no means exhaustive. These substances can be taken alone or in specially prepared combinations:

Argentum nitricum

Arsenicum album

Belladonna

Amyl nitrosum

Calcarea arsenica

Cinchona officinalis

Ignatia

Murex

Nux vomica

Oophorinum

Pulsatilla

Sanguinaria

Selenium

Sepia

Sulphur

Zincum metallicum

The presence of dozens of homeopathic preparations on shelves in groceries, pharmacies, and health food stores is evidence of the widespread interest in this form of medicine. But some experts believe that a premade homeopathic formula is unlikely to match an individual's symptoms or requirements. Guidance is important in selecting a homeopathic remedy, whether it involves a single substance or a combined formulation. As with herbs or prescription drugs, I do not believe that one formula can prove effective for all perimenopausal women, so I advise women to keep this in mind when they are considering homeopathy.

WORKING WITH YOUR HEALTH CARE PROVIDER

Some women who decide to address their perimenopausal health with a herbal or homeopathic approach have the option of working with a naturopathic or homeopathic health care provider or an herbalist. Others have less flexibility—there may not be an expert in these areas near where they live, or the panel of providers from which their insurance coverage permits them to choose may not include an individual who has this expertise. I do encounter lots of women who have a good relationship with their current health care provider, although they are uncertain if he or she will be receptive to trying complementary approaches.

To women who are interested in beginning a dialogue with their health care provider about complementary approaches, I usually recommend these talking points:

+ Begin by talking about your overall treatment goals:

   "I'm most interested in managing hot flashes and headaches."

   "Fatigue is a primary concern for me; I'd like to see what I can do to have the energy I need to move through my days."

   "Anxiety has started to interfere with my work or family life, and I would like to talk about ways to feel calmer and more in control."

   "I've had several bladder infections within the last few months. I would like to get them under control."

+ If your health care provider is not familiar with complementary approaches, it's best to give him or her a clear idea about what you are thinking of trying and why. You'll need to have done your homework. In other words, be specific: say "I would like to try St. John's wort to help with my depression for a month" rather than "I was thinking of trying herbs."

+ Give a clear reason for wanting to try the complementary approach. You don't have to defend or justify your position, but try to articulate the reasoning behind your interest in a particular remedy: "I am more comfortable trying a nondrug remedy to begin with, to see if it helps, before trying a prescription." "I'm not yet ready to begin hormone replacement therapy. I need additional time to evaluate my options, and in the meantime I'm interested in trying black cohosh to see if it will relieve my insomnia."

+ Be prepared to offer backup information or documentation. Journal articles are best—the majority of health care providers would not have time to look through an entire book, and many are unaccustomed to relying on articles in the lay press for information they can use in their practices. You can ask your health care provider if he or she is interested in seeing an article about the particular approach you want to try.

Suppose you've done all these things, but your provider is still resistant, and switching to another provider isn't an option for you now. One of my patients used her strong negotiating skills with her provider. "You would think I'd mentioned snake oil the first time I told him I wanted to see if ginkgo would be useful in counteracting the bouts of forgetfulness I'd been having," said Lila, a 47-year-old who negotiates labor contracts for a major utility company. "He rolled his eyes heavenward and basically said something like, 'It's okay, but you're on your own.' I just came out and asked him what we needed to do to reach an agreement, because I respected him and wanted to continue with him but I also wanted to feel that I had the latitude to make some decisions too. He seemed very surprised when I said that. I guess he just expected that I would either go away and take ginkgo without mentioning it again, or else I'd do what he was recommending, which was to start HRT sooner rather than later."

Lila's provider did agree to make a note in her chart that she was going to try ginkgo: "I had to take the lead and say I'd call him in two months and let him know how it was working, and that I'd come back in in three and look at the whole picture, HRT included, again."

The next time Lila saw her provider, she brought up the subject of black cohosh. "He listened to me quite carefully," she recounted to me, "when I talked about the fact that it has been researched in Europe and that millions of prescriptions for it are written there every year. I said I wanted to give it a try—I wasn't sure if ginkgo was doing the trick for me because I still had times when my mind seemed to be working slowly and I had also noticed more moodiness. He ended up reading the article I gave him, and he did prescribe it for me. I didn't feel like I had browbeaten him or whined, either. I made a solid case," Lila concluded with satisfaction.

PATIENTS AND EDUCATORS

As full partner in her health care, Lila's role in educating her provider by sharing her knowledge about a complementary approach is one many of us in our forties have already assumed or will assume in coming years. With the assertiveness that comes with experience, the ability to know our own minds, and the wisdom about what is right for us, we are changing the path women walk during perimenopause. Whereas women once had little choice but to make this journey as if through a tunnel, guided only by faint light and with no freedom to stray from the course, we walk now in bright daylight, with possibilities for good health nearly as boundless as the reach of the sky above us on a perfect day.

CHAPTER EIGHT

A Decade of
Self-Care

Self-care in the forties is very different from what we did or didn't do in other decades. The old bromides about eating well, exercising, and taking vitamins are completely retooled with new energy, excitement, and creativity. I see a subtle distinction between self-help and self-care, although some might say I am splitting hairs. Self-care places a very healthy and essential emphasis on how we can more fully appreciate and respond to the changes we are going through, taking body, mind, and spirit into account. In our forties we have rich opportunities to embrace change, perhaps more than in any other time of our lives. During this transition, we develop a powerful and integrated philosophy of how to take care of ourselves.

In this chapter we'll look at nurturing and caring for all of ourselves: making conscious decisions to halt our busy pace, seeking relaxation and calm in new ways with ourselves and with other women, moving our bodies in ways that let us enjoy our strength and power, and eating combinations of foods that have a particular ability to nourish our changing nutritional needs. The richly varied textures of life in our forties give us nearly limitless ways to revitalize our bodies and spirits.

Making perimenopause a positive time starts with slowing down long enough to enjoy it. This philosophy flies in the face of the way some women live when they first come to see me with concerns about their perimenopausal changes. Their lives are relentlessly busy, and although the thought of moving at a more deliberate pace can be intriguing, it is also a bit frightening. Connie is the quintessential do-it-all type of woman, holding down a responsible job, coordinating her three children's schedules, volunteering as a Sunday school teacher, and regularly stopping by her parents' home to check on them and bring them books, food, flowers. Now, at 48, the apparent seamlessness of her life was starting to unravel, at least in her eyes.

"I'm having trouble keeping control of my moods," she told me. "There are days when I wake up feeling either depressed or irritable, and the first thing my husband or kids say to me completely rubs me the wrong way." Connie's use of the word *control* was significant—she went on to say that she was struggling not to let her family, friends, and co-workers know that anything was troubling her.

I explained that hormonal shifts could certainly have a role in the mood changes that were alarming her, but I also pointed out that her heavy schedule could contribute to her feelings of being cornered, resentful, or anxious.

"When was the last time you took any time for yourself?" I asked her. "Have you had the chance recently to do something meditative that would replenish and restore you?"

"Well, we did take a vacation last summer."

"Did you plan and organize the whole trip?"

She nodded. The trip had been fun but not exactly restful, she said. Most of the time had been spent on the go, with visits to relatives and long outings every day. "I felt responsible for everything on the trip," she admitted. "I know it sounds strange, but I even worried about the weather."

When I meet a forties woman like Connie who hasn't had a quiet, restorative interlude in her life for a long time, I usually ask her to think back and remember a time (it can be as far back as childhood) when she felt thoroughly relaxed and content. A lot of women wrinkle their brows as they concentrate, because the feeling of being calm or contemplative rather than rushed and busy seems like a very vague memory.

"I used to go fishing with my dad when I was a child," Connie said. "I remember that as such a peaceful time. Sometimes we didn't even talk much, but the silence was very companionable. The sun would filter through the canopy of trees over the stream, and everything was very quiet. I always felt kind of dreamy."

Connie and I talked about what it would take for her to revisit the tranquillity of that time by the stream with her father. "More and more women are fly-fishing as a hobby," I said. "Maybe your next vacation could include some fishing, if you would enjoy that again." In the meantime, since summer was months away, we looked at some immediate steps Connie could take to apply the brakes ever so slowly on the hectic pace of her life.

In our forties we can make our own meditative moments when and where we choose. As some women do, you might want to practice meditation that involves sitting quietly and repeating a favorite word or phrase to empty and calm your mind. At the same time, you can create a vision for yourself that pleases and soothes you. Until Connie could actually get some time away, I suggested that she try taking a few moments to visualize herself beside the shimmering stream where she spent summer days thirty years ago, calling back that calm and safe feeling. "It's best if you can carve out a specific time to visualize yourself in a peaceful place," I suggested.

With women like Connie, who have programmed their thinking to believe that unless they are accomplishing something or getting things done, they are wasting time or being unproductive, the act of stopping and taking time for ourselves doesn't always feel comfortable at first. "But you are accomplishing some extraordinarily important things, physically and emotionally," I said, seeing Connie's raised eyebrows when we talked about meditation and visualization.

"You help your heart by making a conscious decision to reduce your stress — that helps lower your cholesterol. Your body will put out less cortisol, the stress hormone. You'll give yourself a chance to call upon your internal resources, the power at the very center of your being.

You'll build your energy supply back up. Your mind will feel less cluttered because you've made room to think creatively, calmly, and insightfully."

Other women have told me they "don't know how" to relax. In fact the ability to relax is inborn. Every time your body returns your pulse, blood pressure, breathing, heart rate, and adrenaline levels to normal after a stressful incident, you are practicing your innate ability to relax. Sometimes in our forties we just have to retrain ourselves a little to tap into this capability. "Think of taking time to meditate and relax as a different form of discipline," I suggested to Connie, as I often do to women who seem anxious about dedicating time to themselves.

You can start by deciding on one soothing thought or image, as Connie did, seeing herself quietly waiting for fish to pull on her line. Think of the place you would most like to be, and place yourself there for a few moments each day. For Cherie, it was a remote beach in western Ireland she once visited. Doreen made a mental tour through her grandmother's sprawling and comfortable house in the South, long since sold. Ariel insisted that she couldn't think of any image that was relaxing to her at first, but then her face slowly broke into a smile as she said, "I went to Europe one summer when I was in college. I visited the oldest church in Paris on an afternoon in the middle of the week, when it was about a hundred degrees out. Inside it was dark and cool, and there was nobody there. The idea that people had been praying there since the twelfth century was very moving to me, even though I'm not that religious myself. Maybe I should think of myself inside that ancient church once in a while."

The methods for creating stillness and quiet in our minds certainly aren't limited to meditation or visualization. But I often recommend that women consciously take a few quiet moments to reactivate their relaxation response, even if it has lain dormant for years as they charge through life. The activities we can enjoy in our forties, alone or with other people, can also be very meditative and replenishing. Sometimes it's just a matter of putting our own creative spin on something we've always enjoyed.

Pat has loved to read ever since she was a child, but she recently changed her reading list. "I kept up with a lot of professional literature and journals," she told me, "and if I had time to read anything else, it would be history or biography. A friend of mine gave me a book of Jane Kenyon's poems for my birthday — it sat on my shelf for months because I hadn't read poetry since high school English class. My friend never asked me how I liked it, but one day after we had talked on the phone, I took it out and read one of the poems. I just loved it! I finished that book, and then I started reading other women poets, all different voices from different eras. Now I usually read a poem or two before I go to bed. It's a very peaceful way to end my day."

There can be a meditative quality to gardening, sewing, cooking, writing, painting, sculpting, whatever you choose. In fact, your forties can be the perfect time to exercise your creative energy by rekindling former interests or discovering new ones. For several years Andrea had let gardeners take over the care of her flowers because she no longer had time for all the upkeep they needed. When she decided to take more time for herself, she reclaimed one flower bed and dug it up, replanting new flowers in different colors and varieties. "The gardeners know not to touch that section now," she said. "It's mine. Even though it's a small patch of our yard, I could spend hours out there. I had forgotten how much I love turning the dirt over, and how excited I get when the first tender shoots start to come up. I just didn't realize how different it is when someone else does the gardening for me. I always get pleasure from looking at our flowers, but I'm so glad I've started taking care of some of them myself again." I like Andrea's story because it richly illustrates how we need to take care of ourselves in our forties — doing things differently, quite literally planting new seeds, reacquainting ourselves with pleasure in simple and meditative ways, and not allowing others to experience our pleasure for us.

ONE REASON

There is an especially delightful and enriching Native American philosophy that states that every person needs to find one thing, every single day, to be consciously happy about. This very simple meditative technique can work wonders in defusing tension, helping us to live in the moment, and dissolving our resistance to some of the changes we may be experiencing. The marvelous thing about stopping for just a moment to feel happy is that we usually find it difficult to limit our happiness to just one thing—we start to realize that there can be dozens, even hundreds of sources of joy in our lives every day, things we overlook if we don't make a habit of searching for them. The consciously happy moments that women in their forties have shared with me cover a rich range of experiences, from hearing a grandchild's fat chuckle, to smelling fresh coffee in the morning and realizing that the day's possibilities are unlimited, to seeing the elaborate embroidery of a spider's web hung with drops, to watching a hawk soar, to feeling deeply thankful for the love of a spouse, a child, a friend. These small moments of happiness give us time to be attentive to the things we need and appreciate most.

MEDITATIVE MOVEMENT

Meditative movement—combining exercise and meditation? But weren't we just talking about being still? The way we exercise and strengthen our bodies, and our experience of our physical selves, can be deeply meditative in our forties. Sharon found that out when she signed up for a yoga class as a means of reducing her stress level, which had become bothersome for her.

Because Sharon is a strong runner, she signed up for an advanced class, thinking she was fit enough to start with the accelerated group. "How is it?" I asked her.

"I was surprised by how much strength it takes! I'm using muscles I've never used. After two advanced classes, the instructor suggested I switch to the beginning or intermediate class. Actually I was relieved—starting at the beginning is the right place for me. I'm learning about the principles of yoga and the basic poses. That's really building my strength and my breathing capability so I can go on if I want to."

Yoga unites qualities and characteristics especially suitable for women in their forties: strength, flexibility, calmness, serenity, balance, and poise. When we practice yoga, we truly compose ourselves, massaging and shaping our muscles with graceful movement, relaxing and stimulating our minds, bringing comfort and energy to ourselves. The word *yoga* means "union," and indeed our physical grace and spiritual peace are yoked together as we pay attention to deep and often hidden parts of ourselves.

The practice of yoga can bring the flexibility and suppleness we need to move through our changes with power and grace. You can start where you feel comfortable — there is no force, strain, bouncing, or jarring in yoga exercises. The goal is to advance gently at your own pace, never reaching beyond where your body wants you to go, yet feeling the power of your steady progress as your breathing expands, endorphins are released, and your muscles grow stronger. Some of the more advanced yoga poses place weight on your bones, movements that are delicate yet build bone strength and help reduce your risk of osteoporosis.

You may decide to learn about yoga independently, using books or videotapes, and practice in your home. Some women, like Sharon, enjoy the collective calm of a yoga class, the quiet energy in a room with others also realizing their potential for relaxation and strength. A few minutes' daily practice brings a healthy and natural mix of invigoration, energy, balance, and calm to your body, mind, and spirit. The practice of tai chi, a series of slow and carefully disciplined body movements, also provides balance and relaxation to women who choose this quiet and elegant form of exercise. (See appendix B for more information about beginning yoga or tai chi.)

FILLING YOUR DANCE CARD

In her midforties, Olivia started to include fantasy in her exercise routine. "My gym membership had lapsed, but I hardly ever went anyway. I decided I was tired of machines and weights." An ardent Jane Austen fan, she joined a group of people who practiced set dancing, the five movement dances popular in the English countryside in Austen's day. "I love everything about it, the music, the careful quadrilles, the concentration you need to have. You can imagine you're in another century, even though I'm glad I can wear a T-shirt and shorts instead of a dress and petticoats with heavy ruching."

Ballroom and swing dancing are also increasingly popular among people seeking to vary their exercise routines, share time doing something different with people they care about, or bring new friends into their circle. Dance lessons don't have to be formal or expensive — community colleges or city recreation departments frequently offer low-cost classes for beginners and more advanced dancers.

MOVING TOWARD SPIRITUALITY

Mary, who had started walking two days a week with some reluctance, found before too long that her brief strolls were getting longer and that she was actually looking forward to them. "I realized that this is the only time I take for myself," she said, "when I'm not working, paying attention to what my fiancé wants, or getting chores done. My thoughts are less hectic and jumbled because there's nothing to distract me." Angela combines walking and prayer as a meditative form of exercise: "I have a pocket rosary that belonged to my grandmother. It's very worn — she smoothed the surfaces praying for all of us in her family all her life. My own prayers are very different from hers. She knew every saint and observed all the feast days. I keep my petitions simple, praying for strength, peace, and the ability to do the right thing and appreciate what I have. It helps me to stay calm and focused to do that every morning."

Yolanda started a women's African dance group at her church. "We praise and exercise," she said. "We have women of all ages and sizes, moving and bending and shaking and twisting and leaping." She gave a broad laugh. "I work off a lot of tension in that basement." A 47-year-old probation officer who has to work hard not to take home all the trouble she sees every day, she finds release and rejuvenation in dancing with all her heart.

POWERFUL MOVEMENT

As women in our forties, many of us had few exercise and sports options as young girls — we were often on the sidelines as spectators or cheerleaders while the boys played. Many of our mothers didn't make exercise part of their lives either, probably repeating what they had learned: that males are physically active and women are more sedate. My own mother had a Shimmy Shaker in the late 1950s, during the era of all the new automatic appliances. Clocks, can openers, and brooms had become electric — the goal was to save motion and energy, not expend it. Of course, there had to be a contraption that made exercise automatic and effortless. Suburban women like my mother strapped on the belt of their Shimmy Shakers, flipped the switch to the motor, and shook the living daylights out of their backsides. *That* was exercise.

We've also seen the aerobics craze of the 1980s, equally pounding movement and music without discrimination among individual capabilities and goals. I like the wordless comment Lily Tomlin made on aerobics in her performance *The Search for Signs of Intelligent Life in the Universe*. With disco music sounding frantic, almost hysterical, in the background, she rolled her eyes as only she can and moved just her fingers, careful to switch the direction of her frenzied pointing when the beat changed. We've let go of the idea that we have to pound and punish ourselves as exercise, taking a softer and more strengthening approach. Some women prefer to keep a gentle exercise routine, while others work their way gradually toward new forms of exercise once reserved for younger people or men.

Just as women in their forties discover the person inside who does know how to relax, some are also learning that a powerful and competitive athlete is part of their makeup, although perhaps unrecognized until now. In record numbers, women over forty are competing on rowing teams, playing in basketball, baseball, and soccer leagues, swimming in meets, and running track. Many of these midlife athletes never competed seriously in any sport before. Now, instead of watching their husbands or children do it, they are rounding the bases, crossing the finish line, hitting the goal, or swishing the net. With solid builds, powerful muscles, and keenly competitive ideas about winning, these forties women are finding and developing proficiencies they never dreamed they could have.

The time we spend walking, dancing, stretching, or otherwise moving and firming our bodies in ways we enjoy is very liberating. In our forties we feed our souls while we increase our vitality and power. Less concerned about trimming fat, we tune in more to the fitness, stamina, and sensuousness of a toned body.

IT'S ONLY A DECADE: PLAY HARD

We can bring whatever level of drive we want to our work and athletic endeavors, but self-care in our forties also means taking carefree time to play and enjoy ourselves. It is a very feminine trait to be the consummate organizer and efficiency expert, with an unending list of tasks that must be done. As paradoxical as it may be, the forties are the time when we need to be as disciplined about scheduling fun or play as we are about working and attending to other people's needs.

A couple of years ago, I participated in a two-day women's health seminar where the draft agenda was packed with clinical topics that were all very relevant to the audience, which was to be several hundred well-educated and informed women in a major metropolitan city. "When will the women play during this event?" I asked the organizers. At first they looked at me as if I had asked something utterly outlandish. But I explained my position that play has an integral role in our physical and spiritual health. I talked about enhancing the seminar by designating time for humor, relaxation, cups of tea with new-found acquaintances, and music, among other things. We ended up completely revamping the seminar—and it was a great success. The questionnaires women completed after the two days showed that although they were hungry to learn about how their hormones are changing and ways they could gain more control over their own health, they also loved the gift of time to have fun.

Play is whatever you want to make it in your forties; there doesn't have to be a product or an outcome in the end if you don't feel like it. Learning to play might be something like relearning the art of relaxation—it can take some time, and you might feel self-conscious at first, wondering guiltily if anyone is watching you as you do nothing at all, if you please.

Again, the lessons of childhood can teach us something later in life: favorite forms of play from decades ago may have an adult counterpart. One woman I know who loved dolls as a child started spending an occasional leisurely afternoon looking in antique stores, sometimes finding shoes or a ribbon for a doll she was restoring that had belonged to her great-grandmother. "It's like a treasure hunt," she said. A former tree climber heads for an arboretum, a half hour from her home, with a sack lunch and nothing else but the intention to watch the trees mark the seasons' change. A music lover and one-time chorus member parks herself in the listening booth in a music store, switching from opera to hip-hop to country, depending on how she feels. And another woman who loved to "play house" with her sisters sometimes tours real estate open houses in elegant neighborhoods in her community, admiring the architecture, furniture, and decorations and speculating about who lives there.

You can remember your childhood play and bring it back to life as an adult, or even relive it in its purest form, as Jody does when she gets practically elbow deep in modeling clay, finger paints, bubbles, crayons, and glitter with her 6- and 8-year-old nieces. "My sister says they scream with excitement when she tells them I'm coming over," Jody told me. "I don't know who has more fun, though, the girls or me."

I chatted recently with a woman on a plane who was loaded down with official-looking documents and a laptop computer—we both were returning from business trips. As we inquired politely about each other's lives, she mentioned that this had been a fabulous trip. She had looked up two old friends in the city where she had had her business meeting, and on her last evening in town, they laughed and danced and even sang karaoke until two A.M. "I need to do more of that," she told me, looking every bit the buttoned-down professional and most unlike a karaoke singer. "It was so much fun." I would guess that she was in her mid- to late forties, and I could hear the joy in her voice as she talked about playing with two old friends. Her experience was spontaneous, and unexpected pleasure certainly has its own charm. Yet I also strongly urge you to think consciously about playing, even write it on your calendar if you have to, and make sure you have a few relaxing, unstructured, playful hours at least every month. The more we play, the more we learn how good it feels, and the more strongly we will crave time with that carefree aspect of ourselves that helps make us complete.

Nutrition in Our Forties

The forties are a food crossroads, a time when we can free ourselves of the scales, calorie and fat-gram counters, and weight-loss programs with rigidly formulated and expensive meal plans. Instead we turn to a more flexible and integrated way of eating, recognizing that food is a key source of pleasure, comfort, celebration, energy, and strength. Eating well in our forties isn't so much about changing our eating habits as about knowing the full range of our food choices and selecting what we eat with a little more deliberation and thought. I want to review the foods we need more of in our forties, where we could do with less, and which combinations fit best with our changing nutritional requirements. I'll also discuss choosing a nutritional supplement that matches your needs.

THE PLANT ADVANTAGE

When Mary and I sat down to review the food diary she had been keeping for a month, I have to admit that many of the meals she described sounded delicious. But they wouldn't be first on my list to help reach the goal of evening out her mood swings, lessening her menstrual cycle irregularity, and remedying her drop in sex drive, which were the symptoms she most wanted to relieve. We were also aiming to protect her heart, since her father's life ended relatively early with a fatal heart attack.

Mary made many of her decisions about food in restaurants — lunches with clients and fund-raising dinners (where she thought she had no choice about what was served) are a regular part of her calendar. A month earlier, she had decided to try natural hormone replacement therapy to help with her symptoms. Since she chose to use estriol, a form of estrogen that does not provide cardiovascular protection, I also wanted to work more with her on planning meals.

I didn't want to give Mary the impression that choosing healthier foods would mean meals that were dim in color and lacking in flavor and appeal — not at all. We started our conversation by looking at ways she could get more plant-based foods into her diet, particularly phyto-sterols.

Phytosterols are the category of foods that helps to balance our hormonal system by regulating the levels of hormones that are too high and stimulating those that are too low. Phytosterols include foods that contain phytoestrogens, substances that can act like estrogens in the body or affect the way our bodies metabolize this hormone. Adding more of these foods to our meals and snacks during our forties brings benefit to our overall health in addition to minimizing some symptoms of perimenopause.

Soybeans and soy products are rich in compounds that can lower cholesterol, reduce our risk of heart disease, and boost our resistance to certain types of cancer. Eating more soy products during our forties provides us with the added benefit of potentially reducing hot flashes and adding a protein to our diets whose absorption does not leach calcium, as the breakdown of meat and other animal proteins does.

I didn't recommend that Mary begin with soy, mostly because she was unfamiliar with soy foods and would feel more comfortable choosing foods she knew. I suggested that she think more about fruits and vegetables as a way to improve her health. "Many common fruits and vegetables are phytosterols that exert and balance the effects of estrogen and progesterone," I told Mary. "You can add combinations of whole grains and legumes for protein and fiber, and to help fill you up."

I reminded Mary to scan restaurant menus differently and think more in terms of ordering several side dishes, such as a vegetable, a baked potato, a small salad, rice, or beans, rather than an entrée. I also suggested that Mary ask her assistant to call ahead when she was attending a fund-raising luncheon or dinner and request a vegetarian plate. "Almost all banquet halls and hotels are willing to accommodate these requests," I said, "and the special plates are generally much healthier for you. Even at a dinner when everyone is being served at once, you just have to remind the person serving that you requested a special plate, and they'll get it for you."

"Yes, I've seen people do that," Mary said. "I'll just have to think ahead a little more."

"Keep your food diary for another month with your symptom chart. I think you'll see a change in your mood and energy levels, in response to your eating more vegetables and fruit instead of meat and cheese." In another month, Mary came back to say that yes, she did notice a change in the way she felt. "I think it has really made a difference to have a vegetarian dinner whenever I can," she told me. "I used to go home from those events feeling so sluggish and heavy. I thought it was the long-winded speeches, but it was the food!"

This time I suggested that Mary add vanilla-flavored low-fat soy milk to her morning coffee, or put it on whole-grain cereal. One step at a time, she moved toward including other soy foods in her diet. My patient Sharon made time to enjoy cooking and was able to try several soy foods within a month. She too has low-fat soy milk on cereal for breakfast, tosses roasted soy nuts on salads, and "hides" tofu in pasta sauces, on pizza, and in the tuna sandwiches her children eat. Her toddler loves muffins and pancakes, so Sharon varied two of her standard recipes to include soy flour and soy milk. "Nobody in the family even realizes we're eating more healthy foods now than we ever have," she said.

A good daily target amount of isoflavones is about 50 mg. To reach that amount, start with the soy foods that are highest in isoflavones, such as soy milk and tofu. Check the labels, and look for brands that list their isoflavone content. Soy oils and sauces are relatively low in isoflavones.

Another health-enhancing compound found in soy is genistein, a type of isoflavone that may protect against cancer. The soy-rich Asian diet may be one of the primary reasons for significantly lower rates of breast and prostate cancer in Japan and other Asian countries. Researchers are still investigating the cancer-fighting potential of this substance, but indications are very promising that it can block cancerous cell growth or inhibit enzymes that cause malignant cells to divide.

PLANT CHECKS AND BALANCES

With soy and other phytoestrogens, you can't have too much of a good thing. For instance, women like Janice who take black cohosh to alleviate perimenopausal symptoms can also decide to increase their dietary soy if they choose. Like soy, black cohosh has phytoestrogenic effects in the body. The compounds in phytoestrogens have a remarkable ability to occupy estrogen receptors when there is too much of this hormone, and stimulate estrogenic effects when levels are low. We know that deficient estrogen produces its own set of problems — and that overproduction of estrogen is associated with endometrial and breast cancer. But this is not a risk with phytoestrogens. They provide many of the naturally nourishing effects of estrogen, but they are only about two percent as potent as oral estrogens, with none of the side effects.

MORE CALCIUM

Boosting your calcium intake during your forties is a must to protect your bones from weakening as your estrogen levels decline. Because calcium absorption is accelerated by vitamin D, you can combine calcium-rich foods with low-fat milk fortified with vitamin D. Low-fat dairy products are good sources of calcium too, and when Mary and I talked about increasing the number of vegetables on her plate, I mentioned several that have healthy amounts of calcium, from ordinary broccoli and spinach to the less common mustard, dandelion, and collard greens. Lima beans, cabbage, brussels sprouts, green beans, and squash also contain calcium, although in smaller amounts. "Oh boy, a glass of low-fat milk and a bowl of brussels sprouts," Mary said glumly, and I had to laugh. You don't necessarily have to combine calcium-containing vegetables with milk at the same meal if you don't want to, but you'll want to aim for 400 to 800 I.U. of vitamin D daily, along with the 1500 mg of calcium you need.

MORE LIGNANS

"More what?" Mary asked me in disbelief. Found in legumes, grains, and seeds, lignans are a type of fiber that resembles the isoflavones found in soy products. When we eat foods containing lignans, they are converted in the intestines to an estrogenic compound. Lignans may also share estrogen receptor sites, regulating the effects of this hormone.

Flaxseed is very high in lignans. Ground flaxseed or one table-spoon of flaxseed oil added to your diet daily can help regulate heavy menstrual bleeding (flax contains the same "good" prostaglandin found in evening primrose oil), lower your cholesterol, and reduce symptoms of low estrogen. The quality of the flaxseed or flax oil you buy is very important — cold-pressed oil is best, as heat can release toxic substances in flax. Be sure the seeds and oil you choose are very fresh.

MORE OMEGA-3 FATTY ACIDS

Flax also contains omega-3 fatty acids, which have been shown to be helpful in reducing the risk of heart disease. Other good sources of these essential fatty acids are certain types of fish, such as mackerel, herring, tuna, sardines, salmon, and shellfish. Mackerel, herring, sardines, and salmon also double as vitamin D sources, which you can combine with calcium-rich vegetables. But as we'll discuss, animal sources of protein like meat and fish should be enjoyed occasionally by women in their for-ties — plant-based protein is more calcium-sparing and provides the phy-tosterol benefit too.

MORE FREQUENCY

Giving your body a steady supply of healthful foods is one of the best things you can do to keep your blood sugar level constant and avoid worsening perimenopausal symptoms. For Rae, it didn't take long to determine that the irritability and fatigue that were making her feel like her life had turned into chaos were symptoms of starvation as much as perimenopause. "But I do eat," she protested. "I eat a lot."

I pointed to the notes Rae had kept about her food intake for the last ten days. "This says you ate a bagel at nine A.M. yesterday. What time did you get up, and what were you doing until nine?"

Rae is an early riser — she likes to be up before six to have some quiet time before the day begins. Yesterday morning she took her dogs for a walk, folded two loads of laundry, and paid a stack of bills before her husband and son were out of bed. Then she made their lunches, showered and dressed, drove to work, and had the bagel at her desk. She had finished dinner at seven the night before, she said.

"Fourteen hours is a long time to go without food. You were expending energy from the moment you got up without anything to fuel you," I said.

"But I'm not hungry when I wake up," Rae said, something I hear from many women.

"You might not be hungry because you've programmed your body not to expect food until much later. You don't have to sit down for a big breakfast if you don't have the stomach for it, but since you're up so early, try eating something within a half an hour to forty-five minutes of getting up — half an orange and half a piece of wheat toast."

Rae's food diary showed frequent long gaps without food — she would eat something at her desk at one P.M. and then nothing until dinner at six-thirty or seven. "Before we do anything else at all, let's see what happens if you eat three meals and three snacks a day. I have a feeling you'll notice a striking difference in just a short time — more energy and less irritability."

By eating infrequently, Rae was unwittingly sending her body regular alarm signals. When your blood sugar level drops, your body detects that you're in trouble and responds by sending more adrenaline coursing into the blood. These surges of adrenaline (the "fight, fright, and flight" hormone) can turn irritability to rage, anxiety to panic, and tearfulness to a river. Chronically underfed, you can go from feeling merely fatigued to feeling downright lethargic. I wanted to help Rae get a handle on her symptoms before she reached that stage.

Adrenaline also interacts with the hormone progesterone. Research done by Dr. Katharina Dalton in England suggests that adrenaline surges block progesterone receptor sites, preventing the hormone from being used effectively in the body. She theorizes that adrenaline and progesterone "compete," and adrenaline wins out. Adrenaline isn't a good substitution for progesterone in the body; headaches, shakiness, and feelings of anxiety or confusion are associated with adrenaline surges, instead of progesterone's natural anti-anxiety properties. It makes sense to keep your body nourished steadily, just the way you keep gas and oil in your car so it runs properly.

Rae and I reviewed the rest of her food diary, which showed that she ate fairly well but that the timing of her meals was a problem. "Mostly I just forget to eat during the day," she told me. "I get busy, and before I know it, sometimes it's already three o'clock and I haven't had lunch." The simplicity of this solution—eating more often—takes some women by surprise. "That's all I have to do?" they ask, and I often say, "Yes, for now." Rae's point about remembering to eat is a good one, especially if you're unaccustomed to stopping at midmorning, midafternoon, and in the evening to eat something.

"What do you do to remind yourself of other things you need to remember?" I asked Rae. She said, "At work I can send myself an e-mail, and my computer beeps when it's time for a meeting or conference call. I guess I could set it to beep every three hours—that would help me remember."

Other women use lower-tech methods than Rae to remind themselves to eat during the day: they wind a rubber band around the pen they regularly use, turn a picture or other decoration in another direction, or put their car keys, purse, or something else they regularly look for in a different place, so when they have to look elsewhere, they remember to have something to eat. If you're home during the day or on a weekend, you can set a kitchen timer, or follow your toddler's meal and snack schedule if you're taking care of small children who also need to eat regularly.

MORE JOY, MORE TREATS

Your forties are also the time when you can enjoy the foods that build your strength, supply the vitamins and minerals your body requires as your hormones change, and protect you from disease. You need good food and lots of it in this decade, as well as the time to savor it. This is your opportunity, then, to let go of ideas about denying yourself and avoiding "forbidden" foods. Many of us have lived through enough diet plans to know they don't work—in fact, they often damage our health, self-esteem, or both. But in our forties, not only can we eat well with joy and yes, gusto, we can also rest assured that the capability to choose the best foods is part of our own unique wisdom about ourselves.

Sometimes women tell me a certain food is their "weakness." It's often chocolate, as it was with Virginia. She said her clothes were getting tight, she was having frequent headaches, and she often felt depressed, particularly in the last year. She manages a large retail department store that sells plenty of the dark gourmet chocolate she loves.

"Chocolate isn't really a weakness," I said to Virginia. "It's a magnificent treat that's been enjoyed for centuries. But when you're craving chocolate, your body may also be telling you that it needs other things, more magnesium or more of the brain chemical serotonin."

Virginia and I worked out a plan that would have her eat more often and sample more foods with magnesium (cooked soybeans, spinach pasta, a steamed artichoke, brown rice). I didn't suggest that she limit or give up chocolate; I left it up to her to decide if and when she wanted it.

I saw her again a month later after she had been eating frequent small meals. Her mood had improved, she thought. "And my skirts aren't so tight even though I'm eating more." She had had only one headache since our last visit, a relatively mild one. I didn't bring up the issue of chocolate, but she told me with a grin, "I don't have as many gold chocolate wrappers in the bottom of my purse, either." I suspect that the extra sustenance and variety of foods Virginia was trying were helping her to feel more satisfied and less hungry for chocolate.

CONSIDER YOUR SOURCE

Women in their forties are often advised to reduce the amount of protein they eat, but this is really an incomplete recommendation. I suggest tilting the balance more toward plant-based sources of protein and away from animal protein like meat and fish. The key reason to emphasize plant-based protein is that in the process of digesting animal protein, our bodies get rid of much-needed calcium. I'm not saying you should stay away from meat and fish altogether, but when you decide what to have for breakfast, lunch, dinner, and snacks, think plant instead of animal whenever you can.

ONE LONELY APPLE

Once women like Rae understand that eating frequent small meals throughout the day will help them feel more energized and even happier, and that regular nutritious snacks don't mean they'll gain weight, they often ask me exactly what to eat. They're often surprised when I say fruit is a good snack, but not by itself. We derive the most benefit from fruit when we combine it with a whole grain or other source of protein. This combination of foods is metabolized more slowly and evenly, and it won't produce the jump in blood sugar that even a healthy apple can cause. I suggest enjoying fruit with a small handful of toasted soy nuts, half a dozen whole grain crackers, or a thin slice of low-fat cheese.

HEALTHY FAST FOOD FOR FORTIES WOMEN

+ Spin in a blender eight ounces of vanilla-flavored low-fat soy milk, a banana, a handful of peach slices, strawberries, raspberries, or blueberries (fresh or frozen), and five or six ice cubes. This phytoestrogen smoothie will cool you down and give you energy.

+ Fill a whole-grain pita bread cut in half with sprouts, sliced tomatoes, and cucumbers for a different kind of sandwich.

+ Roast a small turkey (it doesn't have to be Thanksgiving) in a roaster bag. It's easy and quicker than traditional methods. Use it as sandwich filling all week.

+ Fill a bag with apples, rice cakes, whole-grain crackers, and roasted soy nuts, to use as snack food. Take it with you to work on Monday morning, so you don't have to remember to bring a snack with you every day.

+ Keep a box of low-salt whole-grain crackers in your glove compartment (it doesn't matter if they freeze or get hot) for times when you are caught in traffic and need a snack. You won't be so hungry, when you get home, that you grab anything you can find.

+ On a cold morning, pour a little apple juice instead of milk on a bowl of Grape-Nuts, and warm it in the microwave. It's a different, delicious, and high-energy breakfast.

- Top a baked potato with low-fat cottage cheese and low-salt salsa.

- Choose something unusual in the produce section, like a mango or a papaya. Squeeze fresh lemon on the fruit for extra tang and flavor.

- Never mind taking time to peel and slice that beautiful kiwi fruit. Just cut it in half, and scoop it out with a spoon. (Remember to enjoy fruit with a small amount of protein to keep your blood sugar level constant.)

HOLD THE IRON

Once you reach your fortieth birthday, you will probably need slightly less iron than you did at other times in your life, about 9 mg a day. It's very important that you get these 9 mg a day, through foods alone or combined with a vitamin/mineral supplement if needed. Spinach and cooked kidney, pinto, and navy beans are good sources of dietary iron. Cooking in an iron skillet also adds a trace amount to what you eat. Symptoms of iron deficiency include fatigue, loss of stamina, and difficulty concentrating. As we've discussed, when estrogen stimulates the lining of the uterus without progesterone adequate to cause it to slough regularly, heavy menstrual bleeding may result. Women experiencing very heavy menstrual periods on a regular basis are wise to have their iron level checked to be sure their blood loss isn't producing anemia.

LESS SPEED

Fast food, with its high salt, fat and sugar content, isn't a healthy or economical choice. But when I talk about "fast food" with perimenopausal women, I'm referring to pace. Many of us bolt our food absentmindedly or on the run, viewing meals as an interruption, something to hurry up and finish, or even an annoyance to shop for and prepare.

Some women also fall into the trap of thinking they have to change the way they eat pronto. As I've said, gradual change usually will be more lasting—introducing new foods like soy one at a time may be the best approach for you. You're directing the experiment—set a pace that is comfortable for you, and allow yourself the freedom to know you won't like everything you try. If I see a woman in her forties whose diet leans toward lots of sweets, fast food, or salty snacks, I generally talk with her not so much about "changing" her diet as about "expanding" it to include more of the foods that will help her to feel well.

I suggest that you take part in the whole experience of eating healthy, colorful, and good-tasting foods, making time to take pleasure and satisfaction in them, either alone or with people whose company you enjoy. Interludes with nourishing meals eaten in a relaxed setting with nurturing company don't need to be reserved for special occasions—you deserve more time to savor them on a regular basis.

SUPPLEMENTING YOUR SELF-CARE

The number of vitamin, mineral, and herb supplements crowding the shelves in drug, health food, and grocery stores can make it difficult to figure out which combination best serves our changing bodies. I discussed herbs that can be helpful during perimenopause in the last chapter—now let's review the process of rounding out and balancing the vitamins and minerals you need.

Supplementation is important in the forties, because most of us don't get every single nutrient we need, every day, from our food. You need at least 1500 mg of calcium daily to keep your bones strong, but other essential ingredients can complement your diet and increase your health and well-being.

Some women prefer to take vitamin, mineral, and herb supplements separately, using several products. This practice is fine, as long as you're careful to take appropriate combinations and amounts. Overall, I favor a simple approach to supplementation: take one good multiple vitamin/mineral supplement each day, along with a calcium citrate supplement. This approach works for me personally for a number of reasons. One, I find it's easy to remember to take my vitamin/mineral and calcium supplements each morning after breakfast. Second, I don't have to spend a lot of time and money shopping for a variety of supplements. Third and most important, I've found a couple of vitamins that work well for me: ProCycle by Cyclin Pharmaceuticals in Madison, Wisconsin, and Optivite by Optimox in Torrance, California. There is also a ProCycle Gold formula with extra calcium that is specially formulated for perimenopausal and menopausal women, but I've found that I feel best when I take ProCycle with a separate calcium supplement.

Choosing a vitamin and mineral supplement doesn't necessarily have to be complicated or difficult. These are the guidelines I recommend to the perimenopausal women I see at my clinic:

- Look carefully at the ingredients, and the percentage of the U.S. Recommended Daily Allowance they provide. U.S. RDA amounts are based on guidelines developed by the FDA.

- Remember that RDAs are general guidelines meant to apply to healthy people — their amounts do not vary according to age and gender. Individual requirements may vary, and at some times, such as during perimenopause or when recovering from illness, more than the RDA of certain nutrients, such as vitamin C or vitamin B_6, may be beneficial. The vitamin/mineral supplement I take, for instance, has higher-than-RDA-levels of the B-complex vitamins: vitamins B_1, B_2, B_6, and B_{12}. I find these B-complex vitamins very helpful in minimizing water retention and depression.

- Vitamin E can also be helpful during perimenopause, regulating estrogen levels and relieving hot flashes, vaginal dryness, and breast soreness. An antioxidant, vitamin E can also provide heart disease protection. (Antioxidants prevent certain molecules from binding to cells and damaging them.) Some women use vitamin E oil as a lubricant directly in the vagina to help with tissue dryness. When taken orally, vitamin E dosages range from 100 to 600 I.U. per day. Vitamin E and iron don't mix, however, so these supplements are not to be taken together.

- Nutrients such beta-carotene, selenium, chromium, potassium, and manganese also have health benefits, although no U.S. RDA has been established for them. I recommend choosing a supplement that includes them rather than taking them individually.

- As I've mentioned, you need at least 1500 mg of calcium per day, more than the U.S. RDA, to maintain strong bones. Calcium citrate is the form that is best absorbed as we grow older and our stomachs produce less of the acid needed to break down calcium.

- Some vitamins can have toxic effects when taken in too-large doses. And the ratio of the vitamins and minerals you take is important—too much of one can counteract the effects of another. That's why I don't suggest randomly mixing individual vitamins and minerals. It's too easy to throw off the essential balance you need to make sure your body absorbs vitamins and minerals properly.

SELF-CARE IS SELF-FULFILLMENT

You truly come into your own in your forties, gaining strength as you change, calling on wisdom you have yet may not have been able to use until you reached this time. Your vision is sharpened and your sensitivity heightened to become aware of all of yourself—your strong body, your calm and centered mind, your joyful spirit. With new maturity you realize that integrated self-care through nutrition, meditation, and playfulness is a powerful act of giving to yourself. Only in this way will you open yourself to all the health, joy, and fulfillment in store for you.

CHAPTER NINE

Changes in the Mirror

*L*ots of women in their forties will talk to me very candidly about the physical and emotional changes they're experiencing: hot flashes, sleepless nights, or difficulty concentrating. But when it comes to changes in the mirror, I notice that very often they bring up these issues last, at the end of our discussion, and often as a joke or an offhand remark. "Things" are happening. Body weight and shape change gradually, yet we're sometimes shocked when we suddenly notice the difference. The face in the mirror may look like a new kind of woman, one we're not quite comfortable with. Girlishness disappears in the forties, and a new maturity informs our appearance.

Lying behind the reticence is usually a mixture of emotions: uneasiness ("Whose body is this?"), and concern about sounding vain or indulgent ("Isn't it silly to worry about a few wrinkles?"). But most of all, I believe many women have an uncertainty about exactly what physical image they're supposed to inhabit now that they've reached their forties. After all, there are no strongly defined cultural standards of attractiveness for women in their forties. That is why I believe we must create them, putting our own signature on what *attractive* means.

In this chapter I want to look at ways in which women of our generation are reversing the social disdain of previous eras for older women. We gain power, wisdom, and beauty as our lives move forward. We measure our worth not by outmoded definitions of sex appeal but by the joy, strength, and peace that we can feel and that our looks can radiate. Yes, our bodies change. But we can understand the physiological reasons for these changes and move toward them with confidence. We'll witness nature's great wisdom and protectiveness in some of our changes, and we'll see ways to celebrate and welcome them instead of using precious energy to struggle against them.

THE SHAPE OF THE FORTIES

As our bodies move toward the biological milestone of menopause, nature prepares us over a period of years, just as she did when we were preadolescents and our bodies began to mature. The changes in appearance are different this time, though, and they can be unsettling if we don't fully understand why they are happening.

Hormone and metabolic changes in this decade result in a different body shape: a waist that looks less pronounced, breasts that seem less firm, hips and thighs that are more rounded and generous than in the past. Women in their forties often think they are gaining weight and try to do battle against their changing shape by cutting their food intake. But as we'll see, eating less doesn't work as a defense mechanism against body changes, and it can in fact exaggerate them.

"When I was younger, my stomach would get puffy every month before my period," Marcia told a discussion group. "But afterward the bloating always went away. Now it sticks out all the time. I look down, and it's like a little tray. I could practically serve you a glass of wine on it." Everyone in the group, a dozen women in their forties, laughed at Marcia's exaggerated description.

I met privately with Marcia a few days later. Her weight has been a sensitive issue for her all her life, and at 46, she views her body's shifts with growing alarm. "I swear I'm not eating any more than I usually do, yet it seems like in the last several months everything is expanding. I feel like I should go on one of those very-low-calorie diets. Maybe now that I'm this age, I just can't eat anything," she said, sounding intensely frustrated.

As Marcia and I talked more, I learned that in fact her weight hadn't changed significantly over the last several months, no more than the usual fluctuations she had had all her life. Yet she was convinced that her hips and thighs were larger—her pants were no longer comfortable. "What's going on?" she asked.

Marcia's body was responding to changes not only in her hormone levels but in her metabolic rate. Researchers don't fully understand why the rate at which we convert food to energy slows down as we age, but it may in fact be part of an intricate relationship between the hormones that govern a host of reproductive and metabolic functions.

"Your body is also changing the way it produces estrogen," I explained to Marcia. "In our younger years, our ovaries are the primary manufacturing sites for two types of estrogen, estradiol and estrone. During perimenopause, as our ovaries produce less of both of these types of estrogen, Mother Nature assigns estrone synthesis to our fat cells. Eventually our ovaries stop producing estrogen completely."

During our perimenopausal years, our fat cells assume this important function that our ovaries once performed. In fact, it is healthy for us to have enough fat cells to synthesize the estrone our bodies require. Later in life, our bodies tend to store fat cells in the abdomen, buttocks, thighs, and upper arms. So the rounded, softer look we acquire is actually the look of health and a sign of nature's protection for our bodies.

"I wasn't thinking about changing hormones," Marcia said. "I just thought I was getting fat." When she completed the clinic's questionnaire about her overall health, I wasn't surprised to see that she had relatively few perimenopausal symptoms—no hot flashes, no vaginal dryness, no depression or loss of libido. In fact, the only change she had observed up until now was that her menstrual cycle was shorter and her periods were lighter.

It's not unusual for women like Marcia, who have softer and rounder figures, to exhibit fewer perimenopausal symptoms. It's as if their additional fat cells are a type of insurance—the estrone they synthesize probably helps to continue the nourishing estrogenic effect even as ovarian function declines. This isn't to suggest that excess weight is healthy. Being seriously overweight elevates the risk of heart disease and other illnesses. Yet Marcia's toying with the idea of a strict diet is at least as unhealthy as gaining extra pounds.

We talked more about Marcia's dismay and her perception that she is "getting fat." She, like many women in their forties, was in her teens or early twenties when the glorification of the seriously underweight body began in earnest with the Twiggy look. Marcia laughed when I brought up Twiggy. "Oh yes, I had the white lipstick, the see-through plastic rain hat, and everything. Never the body, though."

I mention Twiggy as a historical marker — today, in some ways, she looks positively plump compared with the cadaverous models we now see in magazines, on television, and on billboards, so far has the extremism about thinness gone. I don't meet many women in their forties who aspire to the underfed and gaunt look of these models, but the external pressure to be slim is still very real. It was, in fact, our baby boom generation that gave rise to the current idea that women must be thin. While women our age are now taking a lead in dismantling this notion, there are still very strong media messages that slim is elegant, rich, and disciplined while other body shapes are sloppy and lacking in class or even intelligence.

We have the opportunity to turn this perception around. We can replace the goal of an idealized body shape with the conviction that our bodies are changing in the way nature intended, and that our goal is to be fit, strong, and toned rather than slim. I started to suggest that Marcia think more in terms of strength than "fat," but I had barely finished my sentence before she cut me off: "But the waist of my pants is pinching me. That feels fat, not strong, I'm sorry."

"I was getting to that," I continued. "You mentioned that you are considering a very-low-calorie diet. That's a choice you could make, but it wouldn't be the best one for your body and certainly not for your psyche. You probably would take some weight off, but here's what you risk giving up in exchange: your energy and your equilibrium. I'd put money on it that after a few weeks of eating very little, you'd be back here in my office, telling me that you're very tired, that you're bursting into tears for no reason, that you and your husband are at each other's throats because you feel so irritable.

"You have a strong body, Marcia," I continued. "It's working the way nature intended it to. Let's see what we can do to make it even stronger." Marcia said she exercised only occasionally — once in a while she and her husband would walk from their home to the center of their small community. "Can you start doing that two or three times a week?" I asked her. "You'll tone your body, the walk is good for your husband too, and it gives you some extra time together. More regular exercise will also boost your metabolism."

In fact, regular short workouts actually do more to keep our metabolic rate up than less frequent, longer exercise periods. It took Marcia and her husband twenty-five minutes to walk from their house to the center of town. "Doing that three times a week, four when you can, would give you more of a payoff than working out for an hour at the gym once or twice a week," I said.

I also advised Marcia to eat not less but more, with special emphasis on foods with phytosterol effects (see chapter 8). "If you send your body messages that you're going to be giving it less food, it's going to respond by holding on to what it has even longer, and the little you do eat won't be metabolized efficiently," I said.

After only a few weeks of walking regularly and eating more small meals during the day, Marcia found that she felt stronger and more energetic. She decided to find other ways to exercise besides walking that would also be enjoyable and help her to keep fit, so she asked her husband for a different birthday gift: eight sessions with a personal trainer over a month's time. "My boss always talks about her personal trainer, and I used to tune it out as mere boasting. But then I thought about it some more. She's in her sixties, she looks great, and she's totally vigorous," Marcia said. "Maybe the trainer isn't the only reason, but I decided I wanted to give it a try."

The time with the personal trainer was well spent, Marcia told me: "She showed me how to exercise certain muscle groups so my abdomen and arms can be stronger. The sessions were fun, and I saw a lot of progress in only a month."

If the extra attention and specialized training that Marcia enjoyed sound appealing, you can consider working with a personal fitness expert yourself. As with any professional who is going to play a role in your health, investigate the person's background, training, and references carefully before you agree to work with them.

THYROID AND WEIGHT

Marcia needed only a little understanding of why her body felt different to her now, and some basic recommendations on gentle exercise and holistic nourishment to keep her weight stable and provide the energy she needs. But other women have perimenopausal weight changes that are more complex. Sometimes, although they may spend months trying to figure out why they are gaining weight and not feeling well, their thyroid gland is the culprit.

Loretta thought she was going through "the change" even earlier than her mother had. She was 48, and in recent months she had felt unaccountably depressed and fatigued. But most troublesome to her was her seventeen-pound weight gain. During our conversation, we started sorting out her symptoms, which were intertwined. She thought she was depressed and tired because of the weight she had gained, calling it a "vicious circle."

"I'm depressed and lethargic. When I come home from work, I feel like my arms and legs are lead. I don't have energy to do anything. Sometimes I eat all evening long, and the next day I feel even worse."

I asked Loretta if she had noticed changes in her hair and nails. "Not in my nails, but my hair is very dry. That's probably because I haven't been eating right."

I recommended that Loretta have her estrogen and progesterone levels measured so we could take a look at her hormonal profile. The fatigue, depression, and attendant weight gain might be signs of estrogen or progesterone imbalance. I also decided to talk with Loretta's health care provider about having her screened for thyroid problems.

Many symptoms of thyroid deficiency masquerade as symptoms of perimenopause, notably fatigue (often of the leaden variety Loretta described), low-grade headache, weight gain, and depression. Low thyroid is also characterized by dry hair and ridges in the finger- and toenails. Always feeling cold is another marker of thyroid deficiency, as are confusion and painful joints.

During your forties, thyroid screening is not a routine health check, and you and your health care provider can evaluate your symptoms along with any family history of thyroid disease. In Loretta's case, her grandmother had taken thyroid medication, so her health care provider thought it made sense to check her thyroid level. If Loretta's thyroid level turned out to be abnormal, she might need to take supplemental thyroid hormone, which is available in natural and synthetic forms. (Synthroid is a commonly prescribed form of synthetic thyroid; Armour is the natural form of the hormone.)

The best test for thyroid deficiency is the sensitive serum TSH test, a blood test that measures the level of thyroid-stimulating hormone (TSH). This pituitary hormone triggers the production of two other hormones, T_3 and T_4, which are integral in regulating the metabolism. Abnormally high or low TSH levels signal either a thyroid or a pituitary malfunction that may need to be treated with medication. High TSH means your body is deficient in T_4—your body produces extra TSH to try to stimulate what you need. Low TSH means your pituitary gland is not producing enough of this hormone to stimulate the necessary output of T_4.

Loretta's TSH level turned out to be normal, although it was at the low end of the range. So we ruled out thyroid deficiency as the primary cause of her weight gain. Then we looked at her estrogen and progesterone levels, both of which were low. This hormonal imbalance might not have directly caused her weight gain, but I was certain it was a strong influence on her depression and fatigue, with weight gain as a possible ripple effect. We decided to concentrate on bringing her estrogen and progesterone levels back into balance, and since her thyroid was at the low end of the normal range, she would have the sensitive serum TSH test again in six months.

Clearly, seventeen pounds over her weight of a couple of years ago wasn't where Loretta wanted to be. As I had with Marcia, I talked with her about hormone and metabolic changes and her food and exercise options. I discussed the fact that our culture's worship of the thin female body is really very recent, and that goals about body size and weight need to be realistic. The most admired women of the 1940s and 1950s had very full shapes, with strong legs, wide hips, solid arms, and ample breasts. The famous white dress billowing around Marilyn Monroe in that legendary photograph was probably a size 12. Earlier times and other cultures find great beauty and sensuousness in the soft and welcoming look of a round female body.

It's as if part of our society has given away that female sensuousness, the beauty of the round and creamy shapes seen in paintings by Botticelli, Rubens, and Cassatt, replacing it with a look that is bony, rejecting, hard, and unhealthy. We can choose to ignore the messages that insist we be thin and instead heed our own voices, telling us to live comfortably in bodies that are strong, active, and energetic. In our forties, thin doesn't necessarily mean elegant. The desire to be wraithlike can uselessly waste time, energy, and resources that could be expended in much more fulfilling ways.

Public monitoring of certain celebrities' weight provides embarrassing spectacles—they are doing well when they are thin and poorly when their weight balloons. Of course, the celebrities are always women—we witness no such public judgment of men's weight and body size. Women can declare that we won't stand for this measure of our worth, just as we no longer stand for impersonal, standard-brand medical treatment. In a way, the ideal of being thin would have us be weak, powerless, invisible, and ill. We can find our physical and psychological strength by taking proud possession of bodies that have the vitality, energy, and power we need to enjoy our lives.

BREAST CHANGES

Along with rounder, softer hips and thighs and a straighter line where we once may have had the curve of a waist, our breasts change shape during perimenopause. Breast tissue is very sensitive to estrogen, and with estrogen's decline, it loses some of its density and becomes more fatty. Women with full breasts may find that their breasts appear to sag, and smaller-breasted women are often surprised when their breasts seem to become smaller still.

I'm often asked if hormone replacement therapy reverses changes in breast tissue. The answer seems to be that it won't restore the dense tissue we had in our breasts when we were younger. In fact, some women report having uncomfortable cyclical breast changes when they are on HRT, particularly if they are taking synthetic hormones. (But the softer, less dense breast tissue found in older women does make mammograms easier to read and breast changes easier to detect.)

There are several pieces of advice I give to women who are dismayed about their changing breast shape, like Pauline, who worried that her "drooping" breasts signaled that unwelcome changes were in store for the rest of her body. First we have to acknowledge that breast changes may be harder to deal with than some of the other physical changes in perimenopause, because they suggest a loss of youth, sexual appeal, and ability to nurture. I reminded Pauline that when her body began to change in preparation for puberty, breast changes were probably unsettling to her then too. Walk through the halls of a middle or junior high school, and you will see a number of young girls who either walk or dress in a certain way to conceal their developing breasts. The feelings we have in our forties are very different—sadness or poignancy, as opposed to confusion or embarrassment. But the reasons are the same: parts of our bodies are changing, and we need to give ourselves the time to adjust.

It's also important to think about your whole body, without compartmentalizing your breasts or any part of yourself as somehow separate from the rest of you. Your breasts are sexual, yes, but a change at the cellular level doesn't necessarily affect your subjective experience of your sensuality. Even before your breasts changed, they were not your sole means of giving or receiving sexual pleasure, or the single definition of your sensuality, and they won't be after they change either. If you feel regretful or nostalgic about your younger breasts that nursed children, remember that breasts are only one aspect of your deeply feminine side. Your nurturing role has grown now and is becoming more complete with the capabilities that come with wisdom and experience. Nurturing in our forties extends to our creativity in business, art, medicine, science, whatever we choose. We enrich our relationships with children, partners, colleagues, and friends with new honesty and intimacy that couldn't have been ours earlier in our lives because we hadn't experienced enough. Changes in our breasts do signal an important passage, but it is one to celebrate rather than to regret.

The third suggestion I give to women who have concerns like Pauline's is to know that we can refuse to make our breast changes a freighted issue, or to imbue our breasts with more significance than other body parts. One patient of mine returned from a vacation in France where she was struck by the fact that women from 5 to 75 swam and sunbathed topless on the beach, completely unconcerned about the size, shape, or firmness of their breasts. And I have traveled twice to African countries where women do not wear tops at any time. Among the women in several African villages, I remarked on the lack of sexual current surrounding their partial nudity. We can take a cue from other cultures by choosing to regard our breasts as one part of a whole body that is beautifully healthy and resilient, and that has and will continue to be the source of so much pleasure and strength in our lives.

SKIN CHANGES

The first perimenopausal change my grandmother wrote about in her diary some sixty years ago was the fact that her skin looked different, somehow "older" (see chapter 11). For many of us, skin changes get our attention before other signs or symptoms of perimenopause appear. A smooth, unlined look gives way to a face that has broken into a million smiles and been knotted in worry over a million problems, huge and small.

First, let's look at some facts about our skin. The largest organ of the human body, the skin covers nearly seven square feet and includes three layers: the outside layer (epidermis), middle layer (dermis), and bottom layer (hypodermis). This impressive organ accounts for approximately 16 percent of our total body weight and has a remarkable ability to regenerate and heal itself, shedding the surface layer of dead skin cells every day and the outer layer about every twenty-four days.

As we age, fat in the hypodermis starts to disappear, which results in the skin being less soft. No one talks about how wonderful a baby's hypodermis is, but in fact the healthy layer of fat that babies have to protect them accounts for their marvelous velvety skin. At the same time that the hypodermis is changing, glands in the skin's middle layer—the dermis—produce less sebum, a fatty secretion that lubricates the skin and keeps it supple. The dermis is also where collagen, an elasticlike substance, is produced. The mechanism that controls collagen production isn't fully understood, but estrogen is believed to play a stimulating role. As our estrogen levels wane, we have less collagen in the dermis. The top layer—the epidermis—undergoes fewer cellular changes than the two layers beneath it, but we see wrinkles on our skin when the layers no longer fit together.

Our skin also takes longer to replenish itself in our forties. The epidermis has been exposed to sun, wind, or pollutants in the air for more years. When the outer layer of skin is replaced more frequently—as in younger women or in men who remove the outer layer of skin by shaving daily—the skin has fewer lines and perhaps more of a glow.

Skin care in the forties doesn't have to be about expensive cosmetics or so-called antiwrinkle creams, although the occasional facial is good for your skin as well as your stress level. When I see women who want to know what to do about wrinkles, dry skin, or coarse facial hair in their forties, I generally make the following recommendations, in this order:

◆ Joy is the first essential ingredient for healthy and beautiful skin. A woman who radiates happiness in her forties is going to look magnificent, whether she has a few lines in her face or dozens. If you have to search your distant memory to think of the last time you did something that made you truly happy, do whatever it takes to change that now (see chapter 8).

◆ Rest is next—sleep actually wakes up our skin. We've talked about the hormonal influences on perimenopausal sleep disturbances, and ways you can get a more restful night's sleep (see chapter 4). But if you're shortchanging yourself on sleep because you're trying to get more things done on a daily basis, remember that the sleep deficit can show up in sallow, unhealthy-looking skin.

+ Feed your skin. As your hormonal balance changes, you can help restore and stabilize that balance by emphasizing foods that have estrogenic and progesteronelike influences in our bodies. Meals focusing on fresh fruits and vegetables, soy protein, and whole grains will nourish your whole body, and that will show in your skin.

+ Hydrate your skin with plenty of water — at least two quarts a day. Alcohol, on the other hand, has a dehydrating effect and can make the skin look flushed or puffy.

+ Regular exercise will increase your circulation and bring a healthy glow to your face. You can also help maintain smooth, toned skin using facial massage or acupressure. Acupressure involves applying gentle, firm pressure to key points on the face to stimulate circulation and reduce tension. This practice is based on the Chinese principle that essential energy, or *chi*, must flow in even, sustained movements through the body's channels, called meridians. By stimulating *chi*, acupressure can invigorate the face or any other part of the body. You may decide to teach yourself to do simple facial acupressure (see appendix B) or consult a trained acupressurist.

+ It's not new information that the sun is very damaging to our skin, but many women are surprised when I tell them that even full sunblock doesn't fully protect them from the sun's damaging rays. Many women I know have a false sense of security if they've layered on SPF 30 sunblock, thinking they can now spend time in the sun with impunity. But dermatologists now advise using sunblock as only one part of the armament we need against the sun — other skin-shielding tools should include a hat and sunglasses.

+ If the hair on your upper lip and chin has gone from fine and downy to dark and coarse, your testosterone may be out of balance with the estrogen and progesterone your body is producing. During perimenopause, testosterone levels decline slightly. It's not so much the amount of testosterone that is significant, but its ratio to estrogen and progesterone. Testosterone is an androgen, or male sex hormone. Our ovaries produce it, although in significantly smaller amounts than are found in men. During our fully fertile years, the amount of estrogen and progesterone in our bodies may be sufficient to mask testosterone's masculinizing effects, such as coarse facial hair. When the balance changes, increased facial hair or acne can result. Some women choose to have their testosterone levels measured along with their estrogen and progesterone levels. Increasing your estrogen and progesterone levels and bringing them back into balance with testosterone, by means of either lifestyle changes or hormone replacement therapy, can lessen coarse facial hair growth.

✦ Be a wise consumer when it comes to skin products. Many anti-wrinkle and anti-aging preparations are quite expensive, and claims that they remove toxins or rejuvenate cells are false. You have more control over how your skin looks through what you eat and drink and how you feel. If you have a budgeting choice between something that will supposedly make you look better outside, like a skin cream or cosmetic, and something that will replenish your spirit, like a concert, a massage, or a day off for a drive and lunch somewhere gorgeous, I vote for the latter.

SAFEGUARD YOUR SMILE

The forties can be a time when we need to have extra dental work done to replace fillings, caps, or crowns that haven't stood up over time. But some women in their forties need periodontic treatment because early bone loss has led to problems with their teeth and gums. Daily brushing and flossing are routine aspects of good oral hygiene, but we don't always stop to think about our bones in relationship to our teeth and gums. The steps toward strong bones that we talked about in chapter 5 can also help to preserve your smile, saving you from extensive and costly dental work later in life.

CHANGING YOUR IMAGE

The thought of plastic surgery to remove lines, puffiness, or extra flesh on the face or elsewhere makes some women recoil, either because of physical squeamishness or out of a deep-seated objection to the idea that parts of our bodies that have changed should be cut and thrown away. Other women in their forties view plastic surgery as a perfectly reasonable way of availing themselves of medical technology to look and feel better. Still others are somewhere in the middle — they might have plastic surgery if they could afford it or if they could get past their fear of the surgery.

To any woman considering plastic surgery, I advise you follow a careful process before investing time, energy, and money. Start by asking yourself, "Why do I want to do this? To correct a feature I've always disliked? To look younger so I'll feel better about myself? To look younger or otherwise different so I'll be more attractive to someone else? Is there something in my life I'm expecting plastic surgery to fix, such as a troubled marriage, unsatisfying work, or lack of appreciation from my family? Do I have regrets about growing older that I think a different physical appearance will change?"

The French expression *changer la tête* literally means "to change one's head." If a friend tells you you've changed your head, it usually means you have a new haircut or some other new look. The French also say we can *changer les idées*, which means not only changing one's ideas but getting away for a while, gaining a fresh perspective, looking at something differently. Before you "change your head" with plastic surgery, be sure you've put in enough time "changing your ideas," particularly if you're looking at plastic surgery as a way to change the fabric of your life.

Take time to think this decision through carefully, and review your finances. Talk to other women who have had the surgery you're considering, and ask them about their experiences, including the time they needed for recovery. (Some plastic surgery advertising deceptively implies that we can practically "drive through" for certain procedures.) If your friends or family members haven't had plastic surgery (or haven't said so publicly), start mentioning to people that you're thinking about having some surgery done, and ask if they know anyone who has had a similar procedure. You'll usually be referred to people you can ask about their physical and emotional results, and that all-important question, would they do it again? A choice about plastic surgery is best made independent of any advertising, after a careful analysis of your own motives, based on thorough research, and regarding your physical *and* emotional well-being as equal priorities.

How We Look: Changing the Lens

Our perception of our changing bodies has everything to do with how comfortable and serene we feel during perimenopause. Changes in your looks can bring you up short. It's not as if you wake up one day in your forties and find a completely unrecognizable face in the mirror, but every once in a while a realization that you do indeed look different catches you off guard. Allegra, a forties woman with young children who was regularly asked if she is their grandmother, had a spate of these small shocks. "They wear off after a while. I'm used to it now," she told me. "Sometimes I say yes if someone asks if I'm the grandmother, and then they say 'You look so young!' I go right along with them and say thank you. I find it ironic that a choice I've made about when to have children determines if I look young or old."

We can turn and face our changes, acknowledging that it can be hard to leave certain parts of our lives behind but recognizing that it is not artificial standards of beauty we want to preserve. "I've always considered myself a very attractive person," said Jocelyn, who at 49 could still easily make that claim. "I still think I look good" — she acknowledged with a wave of her hand her fit shape and elegant outfit — "but when I was younger, I used to turn heads everywhere I went. My husband used to say that I stopped traffic." Jocelyn couldn't exactly remember the last time everyone fell silent for a moment when she walked into a room. "A few years ago, it dawned on me that I'm not going to create that kind of sensation ever again," she continued. "It was hard to let go of that at first, and I couldn't really figure out why, because I don't place a disproportionate value on that part of myself. I thought about it more and realized that I had some wistfulness about the intensity of my life at that time."

It's natural that Jocelyn would miss the dramatic effect of her traffic-halting looks for a while, but as she nears 50, she looks healthy, stylish, and very happy. She works harder than ever at her job and recently received a professional award. "Everyone in the room was looking at you then," I observed, and Jocelyn laughed. "I didn't think about it, but you're right."

I recently sat in the same room with two women who had very different perspectives about their physical changes. Erin looked and sounded fretful as she said, "I don't like what I see in the mirror. I spend a lot of time putting coverup under my eyes, and I've started to color my hair." This woman actually had few discernible signs of aging, but because she firmly believed "everyone in America wants to look young," she steadfastly resisted growing older. Margo, who was several years older and who had a more mature face, said quietly, "I want to keep every line on my face because I worked so hard to get them." She was raised in a culture where age is associated with wisdom and respect, rather than dread or disdain, and she had taken that philosophy to heart. Her face *was* lined, and her hair was threaded with silver, but she had a peaceful, contented air about her that I wish I could have bottled and passed around to women who fight so hard against changing.

I was genuinely curious when I asked her about her secret for respecting, rather than fearing, her physical changes. "This is the way I'm supposed to look at this point in my life," she told me. "If I looked any other way, I would be out of rhythm with the choreography of my life. I have always believed there is a very elegant and natural order to the way my body and mind change together, and I've tried not to go against it as it unfolds. That's been true all my life."

If we adopt Margo's eloquent and vivid view of life as an exquisitely choreographed dance, we can look at our forties as the time when the movements are very powerful and complete. We can celebrate the fact that we have a transformed sense of wisdom and beauty, and that this womanly grace is something we possess only after living enough years to have earned it.

CHAPTER TEN

Sexuality in the Forties

*M*y full-length mirror is in my bedroom. That's where I stand every morning to check what I'm wearing, appraise how my body looks, and give a last-minute look at my hair and makeup. Both the physical and psychological changes we experience in our forties can have profound effects on our sexuality, and on our experience in the bedroom. Our bodies function differently, which can change our enjoyment of sex. We've also weathered lots of life changes that affect our sex lives.

In this chapter, I'll review how changes in your physiology can play out in the bedroom, and what you can do to stabilize these changes. I'll examine some prevailing attitudes toward sexuality, and how these attitudes shift as we mature. We'll also look at ways to relight the spark, increase your sensual enjoyment (sex being only one aspect of this sensuality), and create feelings of trust and intimacy with your partner.

NOT INTERESTED, THANK YOU

Perimenopausal women, even those in long and satisfying marriages or relationships, often find their interest in sex on the wane. The first possible explanation for a waning sex drive is that our sexual organs and genital tissue are changing. The entire female genitourinary tract is estrogen-dependent tissue. That means that your bladder, urethra, vagina, and external genitalia depend on the presence of an adequate amount of estrogen to stay healthy. With less estrogen to nourish not only vaginal tissue but the muscles controlling the start and stop of urine flow, vaginal dryness, frequent bladder infections, and stress incontinence (urine loss with sneezing, laughing, or coughing) can become problematic during perimenopause.

As estrogen levels decline, the tissues in the vaginal lining can go from forty to four layers thick. Not only do these tissues become thinner, they tend to dry out. The vaginal canal becomes less elastic and actually shortens. This certainly explains why some women feel less inclined to have sex—it hurts. Not only can the vagina feel irritated from too little lubrication, but thinner, drier external genitalia mean that sensation will often be diminished.

The pH of vaginal tissue also changes during perimenopause, which can result in more frequent vaginal infections. It becomes more alkaline, or more basic, and this environment allows more unfriendly bacteria to flourish and cause infection. When bacteria that flourish in the vagina inflame the urethra and bladder, pain and burning with urination, the unpleasant signs of a bladder infection, can result.

If all of this sounds pretty bleak, take heart: it doesn't have to. Less sexual satisfaction is *not* an invariable part of aging. We have many choices about keeping our body parts healthy that are necessary to enjoy sexuality. That was my primary message to Claudia, who was unnerved by some changes in her body she wasn't prepared for.

A woman who said she had always had "an active, healthy sex drive," Claudia was unpleasantly surprised during a long-anticipated weekend away with her husband, and without her two children. "I had looked forward to it for weeks," she said. "We finally had some privacy and time, but my body didn't seem to cooperate. Lovemaking actually hurt. It scared me."

Claudia's husband of fifteen years was very understanding: "He suggested everything from 'Let's try later' to 'What about using hand lotion as a lubricant?' Still, by that time I was mortified."

At 42, Claudia's experience was not unusual. She was surprised and disappointed to find that her physical response to sexual activity was changing, and she wasn't sure why this was happening. She had also had two painful bladder infections within the last six months. I explained that as estrogen declines in our bodies, the amount of moisture or natural lubrication we produce in response to sexual stimulation changes, and that the vagina can become host to bacteria more easily, leaving us much more susceptible to vaginal and bladder infections.

If you've had an experience like Claudia's, or regularly find that intercourse is more uncomfortable than it used to be due to vaginal dryness, don't wait too long to find out what you can do. The genitourinary tract is often the slowest part of the body to respond to treatment for perimenopausal symptoms. If you've had vaginal dryness for a while and haven't done anything to address it yet, don't worry. It's not too late, but an earlier response to this perimenopausal symptom can mean greater and quicker improvement.

I suggested several noninvasive, natural steps that Claudia could take right away to keep her vaginal tissue healthy and avoid chronic bladder infections:

◆ Do Kegel exercises, for overall strengthening of pelvic muscles. You may have done Kegel exercises before as part of childbirth preparation—perimenopause is a perfect time to resume them. By keeping your pelvic muscles strong, you can reduce urine loss if you're having it now, or prevent it in the future. Kegels can be done anywhere—in the car, on the phone, at your desk, whenever you think of it. You simply tighten your pelvic muscles, as if you were trying to keep from urinating, hold for eight to ten seconds (it may take some practice to work up to this long), and release. Repeat at least 20 to 25 times daily.

◆ Try a vaginal lubricant to keep tissue moist. Some women break open vitamin E capsules and place the oil directly in their vagina as a lubricant. Over-the-counter products such as Replens used two to three times per week can also make the vaginal tissue more comfortable. Many women find vitamin E or Replens to be more helpful than other kinds of lubricants, which can reduce sensation for them or their partners.

✦ Acidophilus stabilizes the pH balance in the vagina and can help reduce the number of infections. A beneficial bacteria, acidophilus keeps vaginal flora from becoming too alkaline. Some women douche with plain yogurt, which contains acidophilus; others prefer to take acidophilus orally in capsule form. The Florajen brand is very high in acidophilus content—each tablet contains 16 billion live bacteria.

✦ The herb black cohosh can also help alleviate uncomfortable vaginal dryness. It appears to stimulate the vaginal lining, reducing dryness and atrophy.

Finally, I recommended that Claudia and her husband put another weekend back on the calendar as soon as they could. Not only would rescheduling ease the disappointment Claudia felt, but the reality is that regular sexual stimulation also helps keep vaginal tissue healthy.

HRT and Genitourinary Changes

Hormone replacement therapy often relieves vaginal dryness. But if the combination of hormones in the regimen isn't suitable for an individual woman, vaginal dryness, burning, uncomfortable intercourse, or stress incontinence persist.

As we discussed more fully in chapter 6, HRT regimens frequently include estradiol and estrone, two types of estrogen. A third type of estrogen, estriol, can often relieve vaginal dryness where other types have failed. Frequently called the "weak" or "forgotten" estrogen, estriol has a good track record in relieving genitourinary symptoms such as vaginal dryness and stress incontinence. Estriol is good for hot flashes too.

Although estriol is commonly used in Europe, it isn't made in mass quantities in the United States. Many health care providers are unfamiliar with this natural form of estrogen. Each estriol prescription is compounded individually by a pharmacist as an oral capsule, vaginal cream, vaginal suppository, or topical skin cream or gel. Estriol suppositories are dry and need to be moistened before inserting—they aren't waxy or messy like some vaginal suppositories. Some women prefer to use an estriol skin cream or gel, which is also a prescription medication that must be compounded by a pharmacist.

Dana, a reserved woman with a careful way of speaking, came to see me with this report: "My friends complain about hot flashes, moodiness, and memory lapses. I have none of those problems. What *I* notice is that lovemaking has become painful, and my friends aren't talking about that." She paused for a moment. "Well, I suppose I wouldn't talk about it even if someone did bring it up."

"These are deeply personal issues," I said to Dana. "Many women are uncomfortable talking about their private lives, and besides, it hasn't exactly been common knowledge that these changes can happen in our forties."

As we talked more, Dana said that the vaginal discomfort and dryness didn't happen only during lovemaking. She thought it had started at least a year ago; she is now 47. We talked about her options to manage this symptom—vitamin E or another over-the-counter lubricant and estriol.

After Dana and I discussed her family history and her questions and concerns about HRT, she consulted with her health care provider. Given her symptoms and her overall health profile, neither she nor her healthcare provider thought HRT was necessary for her now. She did, however, decide to try estriol cream, smoothing a very small amount (0.05 mg) on her hands twice a day for thirty consecutive days. She was also going to use vitamin E oil, which can be applied directly to the vagina. As we have discussed, estriol does not affect breast or uterine tissue. Unlike other estrogens, it can be taken without natural progesterone or synthetic progestin, because it does not stimulate the uterine lining. Dana had good results with estriol cream and vitamin E. When I saw her last and asked how she was doing, she said, "There has been a complete turnaround." I took that to be her circumspect way of saying that her vaginal symptoms had improved and, I hope, that she was much more able to enjoy lovemaking again.

SEX DRIVE HORMONES

Testosterone plays a strong role in triggering sexual desire, in both men and women. An androgen, testosterone is produced in males and females, although in much smaller amounts in women. It's important to note here that changes in sexual function are shared by both men and women, although when it comes to midlife transitions, our culture still focuses largely on the female reproductive aspects. But lessening libido and longer arousal time aren't strictly female — the 20-year-old man who needed only five seconds to achieve an erection matures into a 50-year-old who needs thirty seconds and eventually becomes a 70-year-old who may take six minutes or more. Shifts in testosterone levels are part of the changes, as well as shifts in DHEA, sometimes called the "hormone of youth" because it appears in high levels in people under twenty, may also be implicated.

Men too may be surprised by physical or emotional changes that almost seem to sneak up on them, and they may have their own flirtations with anti-aging or youth-enhancing products. Three men I know took the hormone DHEA, allured perhaps by its implied promise of youth and virility. For one of these men, DHEA didn't reverse the aging process as is sometimes claimed. Instead, it led to dangerously elevated levels of testosterone and estradiol. DHEA is a precursor hormone — when it occurs naturally in the body, it turns into other hormones like testosterone and estradiol. In this man's case, DHEA may have spiked his production of other hormones to unhealthy levels. Despite the risks, and without evaluation by a health care provider to see if their DHEA dosage and hormone levels are appropriate, two of the three men decided to keep taking it because they found the idea of staying young and virile so attractive. The male midlife transition is certainly different — less overt and much less widely discussed. As our subjective experience of female sexuality alters and expands in our forties, we should be aware that male physiological and emotional reponses are also steeped in change.

TESTOSTERONE FOR WOMEN

Some women are understandably skeptical when I mention testosterone as a possible aid for perimenopausal loss of libido. They envision themselves developing a deep voice and facial hair, sporting the shoulders of a fullback, and demonstrating aggressive behavior. When testosterone is given in dosages that are too high, or if a woman has trouble tolerating the synthetic form of this hormone, side effects can indeed occur. Testosterone replacement in women should be carefully weighed beforehand and monitored after therapy begins.

As ovarian function changes and hormone production declines, testosterone levels in the female body also drop. We don't see a sharp plunge in testosterone levels — in fact, testosterone drops only slightly in most perimenopausal women. But when the ratio between testosterone and estrogen and progesterone goes out of balance, its effects may either seem more potent or sharply diminished.

It was once believed that taking testosterone would kick anyone's libido into overdrive, but we now know that for women, without estrogen and progesterone present in the proper proportions, adding testosterone alone doesn't do much at all. Women with polycystic ovarian disease, which causes elevated testosterone levels, do not report excess libido — a finding that is sometimes cited as evidence that testosterone is ineffective in treating suppressed libido. However, that view takes only a piece of the picture into account, ignoring the relationship between testosterone, estrogen, and progesterone.

The "Androgens" table on page 199 summarizes some basic facts about testosterone. Like estrogen and progesterone, testosterone is available in natural and synthetic forms. Natural testosterone, which is chemically identical to the testosterone your body produces, can be an option for women who have trouble tolerating the potent synthetic, methyltestosterone. Estratest, which combines estrogen with methyltestosterone, can negatively affect cholesterol and changes liver function in some women.

In the past, testosterone was administered in doses that were much too high for women. These high doses created problems such as facial hair growth, deepening voice, and in some cases irritability. Small doses of testosterone (as little as 0.1 mg of natural testosterone cream can be applied to the hands twice a day with good results), appropriately balanced with estrogen and progesterone, can rekindle sex drive as well as

ANDROGENS

TYPE	BRAND	FORMS	DOSAGE RANGES
SYNTHETIC TESTOSTERONE			
METHYLTESTOSTERONE	ORETON	ORAL TABLET	1.5–2.5 MG/DAY
TESTOSTERONE CYPIONATE	DEPOTESTOSTERONE	INJECTION	
FLUOXYMESTERONE	HALOTESTIN	ORAL TABLET	
SYNTHETIC TESTOSTERONE COMBINED WITH ESTROGEN			
CONJUGATED ESTROGENS WITH METHYLTESTOSTERONE	PREMARIN WITH METHYLTESTOSTERONE	ORAL TABLET	1 TABLET DAILY (CONTAINS 1.25 MG CONJUGATED ESTROGENS W/ 10 MG METHYL-TESTOSTERONE; ALSO AVAILABLE IN HALF-STRENGTH TABLETS)
ESTERIFIED ESTROGEN WITH METHYLTESTOSTERONE	ESTRATEST	ORAL TABLET	1 TABLET DAILY (CONTAINS 1.25 ESTERIFIED ESTROGENS WITH 2.5 MG METHYL-TESTOSTERONE; ALSO AVAILABLE IN HALF-STRENGTH TABLETS)
NATURAL TESTOSTERONE			
NATURAL TESTOSTERONE	NO BRAND NAME — MUST BE COMPOUNDED BY A PHARMACIST	ORAL CAPSULE TOPICAL SKIN CREAM VAGINAL CREAM	1.0–5.0 MG/DAY 0.1–0.5 MG/GM PER DAY 1–2% STRENGTH, TO BE USED 1 TO 2 TIMES WEEKLY

SOURCE: MADISON PHARMACY ASSOCIATES

help build muscle and bone. Women have told me that adding testos-terone to their HRT regimen boosted their energy levels or, as some put it, added "a spark" or a "life force energy."

Testosterone doesn't help all women. Judith told me that several months before, she took testosterone for two weeks to help stimulate a waning sex drive. She wasn't sure if testosterone had an effect on her libido, but she noticed a change in her mood very quickly. She felt, as she described it, "terrible." "After two or three days, I was much more irritable. Irritability doesn't encourage more lovemaking."

As it turned out, Judith was taking more synthetic testosterone than she probably should have. The fact that she was drinking daily may also have contributed to her fatigue and indifference toward sex. Changes in sex drive can often be hard to sort out — where the hormonal component begins and ends, and what role lifestyle or depression may play. Her moods stabilized to some degree after she stopped taking synthetic testosterone, but she was still troubled by her lack of sexual desire.

First, I thought it made sense to measure her current testosterone level in saliva, along with her estrogen and progesterone levels. If her level of testosterone turned out to be below normal, she could consider natural testosterone, since she hadn't responded well to the synthetic testosterone. I also recommended that she cut back on the alcohol by alternating one glass of sparkling water with every glass of wine she drank, to be sure alcohol wasn't a contributing factor to the change in her libido.

Judith's testosterone levels measured 15 pg/ml, which is below the normal range. She was leery of taking testosterone again, but after I explained that the natural form of the hormone is well tolerated and does not produce the side effects associated with the synthetic, she decided to try natural testosterone in vaginal cream form. She used it twice a week for a month and felt a subtle change in her level of desire. "I feel more in balance now," she told me when I saw her next. "I don't have that strange apathy when it comes to sex that I had for months. I've found warmth and closeness with my husband again."

Judith also said she thought that drinking less helped her moods and perhaps her libido as well: "It was a good decision to cut back. The amount I was drinking had crept up without my realizing it. I'm not going to bed with that cloudy feeling in my head from a few glasses of wine anymore. Overall I feel more alert and alive."

WHEN THE MOOD IS RIGHT

When Mary and I had our first meeting about her perimenopausal symptoms, she told me that she sometimes felt like "cringing" when her fiancé was amorous because penetration was painful. Vaginal dryness can make intercourse so uncomfortable that some women may avoid it, even unwittingly. But as I frequently observe in perimenopausal women, Mary's mild aversion toward sex was only partially caused by vaginal dryness. Stressed by a demanding job that left her little time to pay attention to her own needs, she initially came to see me for help with extreme irritability and tension. In our initial discussion about her moods, she readily acknowledged that these feelings also put a real damper on her sex life. She and her fiancé "get into fights that degenerate into a debate on whether I'm being unreasonably volatile or whether he's deliberately trying to drive me crazy. Then we're both so angry and tense that neither of us has any affection to show the other."

A few months later, Mary's story was different. She had been using natural progesterone to help with her anxiety, and estriol for her vaginal dryness and drop in sex drive. At the same time, she instituted two very new practices—walking at least twice a week while squeezing her hand-held "stress balls" instead of a cell phone, and passing on rich restaurant meals in favor of vegetables, fruits, and grains, to help restore hormonal balance. It wasn't long before she saw a difference in her outlook.

"I perceived the change at a very visceral level right away, within days, as if a knot in my stomach dissolved," Mary said. "More gradually I noticed that I could be more relaxed sexually, too, probably because I didn't have the vaginal dryness and burning, but also because I didn't feel so frantic about my work and my life." Her testosterone levels were also low, but in her case regulating her estrogen and progesterone levels and incorporating some important lifestyle changes had made a distinct difference in the way she felt physically and emotionally.

DEPRESSION AND LOSS OF LIBIDO

Lack of interest in sex is commonly regarded as a sign of depression, but in perimenopausal women suppressed libido and depression are complex bedfellows. Depression and lack of libido may both be signs of a hormonal imbalance, but the hormonal component is often overlooked, under the mistaken assumption that women in their forties are too young for "the change." Women who are prescribed an antidepressant may find their interest in sex more remote than ever. That was true of Caroline, who at 48 said she had little sexual desire and that when she did make love, she found the experience curiously unsatisfying.

Caroline's feelings of depression might have been independent of hormonal changes, but I wanted to make sure we had the whole picture. At the end of our discussion, I suggested that she talk with her health care provider about three issues:

+ Hormone measurement. Measuring the saliva or blood levels of Caroline's estrogen, progesterone, and testosterone would give us more information about other possible influences on her lack of libido and depression.

+ Alternative medication for her depression. Caroline was taking a selective serotonin reuptake inhibitor (SSRI). These medications can be very effective in managing depression, but some women report side effects of decreased libido or difficulty reaching orgasm. Switching to a different SSRI sometimes helps, but some women prefer to try the herb St. John's wort. This herb also acts on serotonin levels but does not have side effects.

+ Referral for counseling. Caroline said she "loved her husband dearly" but also had feelings of lingering disappointment about his erratic career and the financial burden that his spotty work record had placed on her. I could see this was a difficult subject for Caroline, and I thought it would help her to explore it more fully, initially in one-on-one counseling and perhaps later with her husband in joint counseling.

I'D RATHER TAKE A NAP

The simple matter of energy, or lack of it, can put a damper on even the most fulfilling sexual relationship. Lack of sleep and an overabundance of worries can put a sexual rendezvous at the very bottom of your list of priorities. When we're in our forties, those thieves of our energy can take many shapes. Hormonal changes can produce sleep disturbances that leave us feeling gritty-eyed and depressed during the day. Come night-time, we're mainly hoping not to have a rerun of last night's insomnia and maybe we're not even thinking of sex. Some of us are mothers of newborns, dealing with sleep deprivation and hormonal shifts related to breast-feeding. Others lie awake tossing and turning because our teen-ager is out with the car.

The successes, disappointments, and rigors of our jobs weigh in heavily during our forties, keeping us awake at night or draining us during the day. Janice was often sleepless worrying about her mother, whose forgetfulness made her wonder if she had turned off the stove, or closed and locked the front door. The combustible mix of work and family pressures can keep us exhausted, preoccupied, or both, dulling the edge of sexual desire.

Having enough stamina to enjoy sex starts first and foremost with having enough energy for ourselves. A nourished and rested body is more able to respond to everything life promises—sex, excitement, change, stress, opportunity, challenge, and difficulty. Good food and adequate sleep may not sound like aphrodisiacs, but if either is missing from your life, nutrition and rest can bring balance into your life and more joy to your bedroom. (See chapters 4 and 8 for a discussion of how.)

It's equally essential to provide sustenance for your soul and spend time playing, meditating, relaxing, or doing nothing at all if you choose. You can stretch yourself to the maximum in your forties, but I propose you turn your attention instead to your limitless opportunities to replenish yourself. You can actively trade a frazzled, depleted self for one that is reposed, peaceful, and more open to pleasure of all kinds.

SEXUAL LIFE OF THE MIND

Some of the obstacles to the full enjoyment of sexuality can be addressed relatively straightforwardly: restoring hormonal balance to replenish vaginal tissue, finding the right combination of food, exercise, and relaxation that will give us enough energy to be sexual, and adding herbs or hormones to help with mood changes when depression or irritability gets in the way of an active and healthy sex life.

But in our forties, as our view of ourselves changes, the nature of our relationships also takes on a different cast, and many of our attitudes about our sexuality are also reformed. Some of us grew up with either little or no information about sexuality, or with veiled messages that sex was at worst embarrassing and at best simply not spoken about. Many women of our age experienced tremendous pendulum swings in social attitudes about sexual behavior. Parental lessons about modesty or good behavior may have given way to sexual experimentation and having multiple partners. I see women who have regrets about their past sexual behavior, some because they wish they had been more discriminating, like Lenore, and some who wish they had experimented more freely, like Julie.

"The thrill of being chosen by men was a very heady experience when I was younger," Lenore said. "I thought my own value rose in proportion to the number of men pursuing me. If I had it to do over, I would have valued more things about myself than my appeal to men. I would have focused on my studies and my career when I was in college, and more on my kids when they were young, right after I got divorced."

Lenore's daughter was 14. "I talk to her a lot about respecting herself and respecting her body. I'm trying to give her messages that will help her develop self-confidence. I've been honest in telling her that I've chosen badly in the past by defining myself in terms of my appeal to men or by placing their approval of me above other more important things. I don't go into detail, but I still wish I didn't have to be guarded when talking about that part of my life."

Lenore mixed strength and pragmatism into her view of what she described as "sexual acting out" in the past. "I'm not trying to rewrite my history, because I know I can't," she said. "But I decided a long time ago that I wanted to give my daughter very careful guidance and explicit reinforcement about her own self-worth, not from the standpoint of learning from my mistakes, but to present myself as a concerned and caring mother who has something important to share."

Julie, on the other hand, told me she "sat out the sexual revolution" and occasionally wondered what she missed. "I was shy as a child, and that continued through adolescence and young adulthood. I had very few relationships before I met my husband, and only one was sexual. My girlfriends had lots of boyfriends, different ones every few weeks, it seemed. That kind of lifestyle wasn't for me, but sometimes I wonder what it was like."

Julie's fleeting thoughts about having missed something in the past might have more to do with an absence she feels now, at age 46. "That could be," she agreed. "I grew up very fast and assumed a lot of responsibility at an early age because both of my parents worked. I was already pretty old for my age in my midteens. No one forced me to help with my younger brothers and the house—it was just my personality."

The serious, responsible side of Julie's nature has served her well as an adult, but I suggested that she take time now, in her forties, to explore what it would feel like to be more playful and carefree. "I'm not talking about sexual abandon," I said, seeing her face. "It's just that you didn't have the chance when you were younger to put down your cares. You might find that very freeing now."

For many women in their forties, the relationship between sex and conception also changes dramatically. You may have spent your twenties or thirties carefully avoiding pregnancy until you were ready to start your family. If your family is complete now, the experience of sex shifts from an emphasis on making babies toward an emphasis on sharing intimacy and affection. For plenty of other women in their forties, sex and conception are still inextricably linked—they have decided it is time for their first baby, or for another one even if their children are older now. Still other women in their forties have been trying for years to conceive a first child; for them sexuality is intermingled with disappointment and sorrow.

SINGLE LIFE IN THE FORTIES

Our forties are often a time when many women find themselves newly single. "All the rules have changed," exclaimed Christine, a year after ending her eighteen-year marriage in divorce. "I feel like Rip Van Winkle, coming awake in a different century."

Women like Christine who face being single in their forties, whether they are widowed or divorced, may be terrified at the thought of dating again, let alone entering into a serious long-term relationship. When they dated as young women, the specter of AIDS or other sexually transmitted diseases never entered their minds. They may fear that their opportunities for love are now limited because they are not as young as they used to be. And relationships can be much more complicated when shared custody of children and changes in financial status are part of them.

"Take a few steps back, and think about your own needs now," I suggested to Christine. "You have an opportunity to discover things about yourself at this time in your life that you may have ignored before, or not had the chance to develop."

Her loneliness and feelings of insecurity, I suggested, are a natural outcome after ending a long marriage or relationship. "The company of friends can be very healing while you adjust to life without your ex-husband. Companionship and support are important for you now," I said. "You'll decide when the ground underneath you feels solid enough again to think about another relationship. You'll be the only one who will know when that time has come."

Christine's marriage had been troubled for several years before she and her husband decided to divorce, so in the aftermath, shock wasn't among the feelings she struggled with. Sarah, however, still finds herself stunned and disbelieving two years after her husband's sudden death. "I never dreamed I would be by myself at forty-four. Of course I knew about all the things that can rock a marriage, but death at this time in my life? I was utterly unprepared.

"I can't tell you how many people have said to me, 'Don't worry, you're young, you can remarry.' I know they meant well, but they have no idea what a stinging statement that is. I don't *want* to remarry. I wanted to live out a long life with my husband and get very old with him." She sighed. "Now I have friends trying to fix me up with single men."

"Do you meet them?" I asked her.

"I did, a few times. Then I decided not to anymore because I always felt so depressed afterward. I'm not sure why, because a couple of them seemed perfectly nice."

"When you're ready to go out again, perhaps you can consider meeting the men your friends suggest more as part of enlarging your circle," I said. "See if you can just enjoy talking with someone new, telling him about yourself, solely for the purpose of having a good time. You don't have to think beyond the moment if you don't want to. It might feel less depressing that way, and less like every date is a poor stand-in for the husband you still miss so much."

Christine and Sarah are single in their forties for very different reasons; one has some feelings of relief while the other is still struggling to get past devastation. Yet I made three similar suggestions to both of them: "First, be very protective of your physical health. I would tell you that even if you weren't in the middle of adjusting to an enormous life change, but it's doubly important now. Then, take the time you need to crystallize a very clear idea about what you want, not necessarily with respect to relationships but for your whole life — what you need for security, fulfillment, and happiness. Finally, remember that the keys to your fulfillment are within your own energy, creativity, and capacity for healing and renewal. When and if you're ready, you can bring all those qualities to the type of relationship that will be right for you."

SENSUALITY AND INTIMACY

The forties are a time when we can make sense of shifting and sometimes conflicting attitudes about sexuality, by seeking full expression of our sensuality. Sexuality is just one of many pleasures we give and receive. Voluptuousness in our forties makes the true definition of the word come alive — indulgence of luxury, enjoyment, and sensual pleasure.

"What do I know from indulgence or luxury?" Bonnie asked me. "I have too much to do, and not enough time or money." That was my point exactly — the frenetic busy-ness of many of our lives keeps us away from ourselves, from the expression of our sensual side.

"Maybe we're defining things differently," I said to Bonnie. "I don't mean luxuries that have to be expensive, or indulgence in a negative sense that's lazy or selfish. I'm talking about luxuries like having time to yourself, or having intimate, meaningful time with someone you care about, where the goal is to be together, without expectations about getting something done."

The awakening of your sensual side can happen through whatever combination of touch, smell, taste, sound, and vision you choose. Maureen enrolled in a sculpting class at a community college, intending to take some time for herself and to ease her stress level. But she found that kneading and shaping the clay, rolling it beneath her fingers, pounding it with her fists, was a sensual experience that left her not only more relaxed but energized at the same time. Andrea, who started gardening again after a long hiatus, had a similar sensual experience as she worked the warm soil and breathed the scent of the peonies and dahlias. "When I was growing up there was an older woman in our neighborhood who used to garden at night. She grew potatoes in straw. Everyone claimed that she gardened in the nude, although no one had actually seen her," Andrea told me. "I don't know what made her come to mind recently. I probably hadn't thought about her for twenty-five years. But there's something very appealing about the idea of gardening on a warm night with no clothes on. I just might try it."

Sheila created a ritual for herself that soothes her and enlivens her senses: she listens to a favorite Bach piece, lights some soft candles, and bathes in scented oil. Afterward she dresses in an outfit of soft fabric and subtle colors she loves. She sometimes performs this ritual before meeting a friend at a café or museum, but she often does it just to relax by herself at home or before going somewhere alone. "I feel like I really own my body when I'm finished," she says. "My blood is humming, and my mind is refreshed."

Mindy delights in touch, smell, and taste when she devotes a Saturday each month to baking and freezing loaves of crusty whole-wheat bread. "I play out lots of emotion as I shape the dough," she said. "The smell fills the whole house, and when the bread is done, I cut a thick heel for myself and have it with tea. My family looks forward to those Saturdays as much as I do."

I often talk with women in their forties who yearn for a kind of intimacy and closeness that is nonsexual — for more expressions of caring from their husbands or partners. I always ask what these expressions of caring would look like, or what would define such intimacy. I get a range of responses, some of which are completely unrelated to sex:

"Being hugged, tenderly kissed and held, not just as part of making love."

"Reaching for my hand in public."

"Whispering something loving to me instead of just pressing up against me when he wants to have sex."

"Calling me once in a while during the day to ask if there's anything he can do on his way home, or just to say he's thinking about me."

"Listening to me if I'm upset. Just being able to say what's on my mind is so much more helpful than being told 'It will be okay,' or worse, 'Calm down.'"

"Planning an evening out—getting the tickets, making the reservation, whatever, getting the babysitter—so all I have to do is show up and enjoy his company. We never get out unless I arrange everything."

My next question is always the same: "Have you asked for any of these things?"

"Well, not exactly," Helene told me. She was the woman who wished her husband's show of desire were a little more expressive than pressing against her. The parallels aren't exact, but in some ways achieving the intimacy we seek is similar to getting the health care we need: both depend on our knowing what we want and asking for it, very specifically, without being critical or apologetic. "The next time your husband initiates sex without a word, can you say something like 'I'd be so happy to hear you tell me you love me'?" I asked.

Sometimes demonstrating the kind of closeness we would like him to show us helps too. I suggested that Aileen take her husband's hand often in public instead of waiting in vain for him to be publicly affectionate toward her. She was gratified when he reciprocated, stealing an arm around her shoulders or waist. Corinne also decided to take the lead: she picked up the phone and called her husband for a brief hello while he was at work a few times. "The first time, he barked, 'What's wrong?'" she said. "Now he seems genuinely happy to hear my voice. The other day I asked him to call me if he got a chance, and he did. We don't talk long, but the tone is always very warm. I love that. Before we started talking occasionally during the day, it seemed like our discussions were all business."

Deepening your intimacy with your partner requires a certain clarity about what you expect; it also means you have to take the time, apart from chores, bills, jobs, children, in-laws, and other "business," to focus on your commitment to the person you care about without distraction. But our sensuality and passion are expanded in our forties—it becomes more than sexual feelings or acts, more about intimacy with others, involving a show of tenderness and trust born of confidence about our own strengths and needs. Our definition of romance matures: a spray of roses or a bottle of champagne seems less romantically charged than an evening spent intertwined on the sofa.

As you both adjust to physical changes during your forties, you and your partner can also use your broadened outlook on romance to your advantage:

- ✦ Plan regular, quiet, intimate times with your partner when the rest of the family is elsewhere, and the phone, television, beeper, and computer are turned off.

- ✦ Listen to favorite music together, or if one or both of you plays a musical instrument, perform a recital just for your mate.

- ✦ Take a look at photographs of your early days together, and describe your memories to each other.

- ✦ Read aloud to the person you love, or ask him to read to you as you cuddle. Short stories or poems are well suited for one session, but you might even decide to read a novel together in installments, one section at a time.

- ✦ Find a comfortable place to stretch out, and massage each other's feet. Revel in the sensuous, comforting touch.

- ✦ Talk about the time when you met and were getting to know each other. It's lovely to tell, and to hear about, the characteristics that drew you to each other.

You may have slowed your pace, yes, but you've also deepened your appreciation of the many meaningful ways you can be together with someone you love. Intimacy is there for you in your forties, waiting for you to recognize what it is and move deliberately toward it.

CHAPTER ELEVEN

Empty Nest/
Full Nest

*W*e're living in a truly amazing time in our history: while some women in their forties are seeing their children out into the world, others are having their first babies or caring for young toddlers at home. The predictability of the 1950s, where women pretty much stuck to a timetable — or were pressured to do so — has given way to a vast flexibility in reproductive lifestyle.

Today, when it comes to childbearing, everything under the sun is possible, which includes negative as well as positive developments. Not only are women having babies throughout their fertility cycle, but they, with their partners, are grappling with a crisis in fertility that has galvanized the technological world.

In response, fetuses are stimulated into being in laboratories and are born and kept alive far earlier than was ever possible before. The viable weight for premature babies is becoming smaller and smaller. Reproduction in our time has truly become a mosaic of possibilities.

In this changed world, our emotional and hormonal responses to childbirth and childrearing can be overwhelming and profoundly confusing. As we break the molds, we find ourselves without role models to guide us. Whether we have recently given birth or are preparing for our grown children to leave, we face psychological and biological challenges, no matter what our family constellation looks like.

Not only do we have nests with our families in the forties, but if we have parents or other relatives who need more help and care, we must often pay increasing attention to the nest that gave us our start. The competing demands of two generations place additional emotional and financial demands on women sandwiched between them. In this chapter we'll discuss the keys to finding balance as our families take different shapes, and how your own changes can help you respond to conflicting needs with clear-eyed discernment and equanimity.

NEVER ALONE, YET LONELY

"I was forty when I had my daughter, and I was overjoyed because I didn't have an easy time getting pregnant. But it's the craziest thing since she was born. I never have five minutes to myself, but I find myself feeling lonely a lot," said Anne-Marie.

"The feeling started shortly after she was born. I'm the youngest in my family, so it was literally forty years since my own mother had a baby, and so much has changed. I felt like we didn't have as much to share as we did before. My mother isn't really old-fashioned, but she thinks it's masochistic to go through childbirth without medication, and she couldn't believe I wasn't sterilizing all my bottles. Don't get me wrong, she wasn't judgmental or critical — we just occupy different generations. But it might as well be different planets."

Differences between raising children now and forty years ago weren't the only reason for Anne-Marie's loneliness. "I know lots of women are having babies later in life, but where are they? I joined a mothers' group and an exercise class, but all the moms were fifteen to twenty years younger than me. They all looked so energetic and happy, and I felt very bedraggled and tired in comparison."

Now 42 with a toddler who keeps her running every minute, Anne-Marie experiences fatigue as a natural outgrowth of meeting a demanding two-year-old's needs. But perimenopausal changes may also account for her lower energy levels. And although she calls it loneliness, some women of perimenopausal age experience feelings of depression that seem unrelated to any external cause. I suggested that her situation warranted taking a closer look. Anne-Marie needed help sorting out her feelings of loneliness and fatigue to determine whether they were physical, psychological, or a combination of both.

I started by asking Anne-Marie to describe her typical day, and as I expected, she said she started early and ended late, amusing, entertaining, and caring for Sophie during her waking hours, and doing chores while she slept. For an hour or two after Sophie went to bed in the evening, Anne-Marie got ready for the next day, straightening the house, doing laundry, preparing meals, or paying bills. As she had said even before giving me this rundown, Anne-Marie's schedule didn't include time for herself. I noticed that while Anne-Marie spent a good deal of time and energy making sure Sophie ate well, she herself ate haphazardly and paid little attention to what she was putting in her mouth.

Anne-Marie also talked about her role as a mother and the conflicting feelings she had on most days. She had taken a hiatus from the world of investment banking, where she had worked from the time she finished her education until having the baby two years ago. "I'm happy to have the time to be home with Sophie without a lot of financial pressure," she told me. "She's very bonded to me, and I've tried to teach her a lot. But sometimes I do get bored and restless. It's hard to think of endless ways to keep her attention, and there are times when I think I can't possibly read the same book to her again. I miss adult company, and I can't really keep up with industry trends. I used to stack up *The Wall Street Journal*, thinking I'd get to them, but a few months ago I threw away a huge pile and canceled my subscription. There's just no time. I also worry that by the time Sophie goes to school and I want to go back to work, it will be hard to achieve the seniority and salary I worked for years to attain."

I recommended that Anne-Marie take four steps right away:

✦ Give herself a healthy dose of credit. "You're bringing a lot of patience and dedication to your daughter's life," I said. "It's not always easy to take care of a toddler, but you're achieving two very important things: building a safe and secure environment that will serve her all her life, and stockpiling memories for yourself that you'll treasure forever."

+ Put herself on her daughter's feeding schedule. "Eat more regularly during the day," I advised Anne-Marie. "When your daughter has a meal or a snack, have some fruit and crackers or a half a sandwich too. You could be tired from not eating enough of the right things." Anne-Marie told me that in the past two years, she had been very concerned about gaining weight. "I try to eat very little during the day because I don't want to start snacking and putting on weight," she said. I explained that refueling her body at regular intervals with a nutritious snack wouldn't make her gain weight but would help her counteract her depleted and drained feeling.

+ Take time for herself. Anne-Marie took motherhood very seriously, but I reminded her that her job description included taking care of herself. "Instead of doing chores while Sophie naps," I suggested, "have a babysitter come for an hour or two, and get out by yourself. You could go to a bookstore or to the library to catch up on *The Wall Street Journal* or anywhere you like that would give you a break and some stimulation."

+ Be alone with a friend to combat loneliness. "Schedule a lunch date with a friend or someone you used to work with," I said. "You can catch up on professional news if you like, or just take time to finish a meal and a conversation without interruptions." Anne-Marie hesitated before replying. "That would be a luxury," she said. "No, it's essential," I said. "I'd write you a prescription for it if I could."

Anne-Marie agreed to try these four steps over the next month. "If there's no change in your feelings of fatigue and loneliness, I'll recommend that we evaluate your hormone profile to see if changes in estrogen, progesterone, or testosterone are also influencing your feelings." I had a feeling, though, that as a forties mother striving for excellence as a parent just as she had as a banker, Anne-Marie had placed her own needs lowest in the hierarchy of needs she had to meet every day.

I actually didn't see Anne-Marie until six weeks later. "I've been so busy," she said. Busy with games and puzzles, yes, but she had also reconnected with some of her colleagues. She looked happier and more animated as she told me her former co-workers were interested in having her work as a consultant on a couple of special projects. "I could do the work from home and make my own hours and terms."

"Is your energy level any better?" I asked.

"I think it is. It took me a couple of weeks to get started eating meals and snacks with Sophie — I had to convince myself that I wasn't just stuffing myself. Actually, it's been good for both of us. Sometimes I'd give her cookies as snacks, but now we're both eating more fruit, lightly steamed vegetables, and bites of low-fat cheese. Her appetite is better, and I'm not feeling like I need a nap as often."

In two subsequent discussions I had with Anne-Marie, we laid more of the foundation for integrating her physical, emotional, and spiritual needs into the day-to-day tasks involved in raising her small child. "There's so much fun ahead as your daughter grows and develops," I said. "You'll get the full measure of enjoyment from these years if you preserve *your* physical health as carefully as you're looking after your daughter's. And by making sure you take time for yourself to recharge your energy and pursue your professional and personal interests, your own growth will continue." It's easy to lose track of our own needs in the face of everything it takes to keep our children safe, amused, nourished, clean, rested, and stimulated, but I urged Anne-Marie to think of her self-care plan during this decade as a form of protection not unlike her daughter's immunizations. The reserves of strength and peace of mind we build in our forties will come back to us as we savor the present and greet the future.

Can *I* Do It?

The decade of the forties is a time when some women decide to have a baby, either for the first time or to complete a family they started many years ago, while others build an extended family with a different spouse. "I'd like to have another baby, but I just don't know if I can do it," said

Maggie wearily. Recently remarried at 42, she has a 12-year-old son and a 15-year-old daughter. "My sleep is always restless, and I wake up exhausted. When I think about having to tend to an infant in the middle of the night besides, I start to think I'm nuts even to consider it."

Yes, Maggie thinks about her new "blended" family, her job, her ex-husband, and her new spouse as she lies awake. But her late-night wakefulness may also have a hormonal component that is heightened by the changes and challenges in her life. As our estrogen levels decline, the relationship between this hormone and neurotransmitters can be thrown off. The neurotransmitter serotonin plays an important role in governing our patterns of sleeping and waking. If our levels of estrogen and serotonin are seesawing up and down, fitful sleep may result.

Making decisions large and small can seem like a very tangled process when you don't have enough sleep. "Let's see if we can get your sleeplessness under control first," I suggested to Maggie. "There may not be a way to have absolutely clear feelings about another baby, because that's a complex issue, but I'd like to see if we can stabilize your sleep patterns."

Maggie was interested in trying valerian root, a herb used for its calming properties and to promote sleep (see chapter 8). I also suggested that she begin and end her day with a series of progressive relaxation exercises that can be done in bed — tensing a group of muscles and releasing them, working up or down from head to toe until the whole body is relaxed.

Women like Maggie who wrestle with the decision about having a baby in their forties may not only have to grapple with their own conflicting feelings but contend with comments and judgments from friends, family, colleagues, or in some cases, their spouse. "People act like I'm a hundred instead of forty-three when I talk about wanting another baby," said Alison with some resentment. "They say 'At your age?' or 'Isn't two enough?'" The mother of two daughters, 16 and 20, Alison says she'll approach motherhood differently this time. "I've learned that children need more time and attention and fewer material things," she says. "And I'd be less inclined to make this baby the focus of my whole life, so that everything else came second, including my marriage and myself."

Women like Maggie and Alison who yearn for a baby in their forties may also want another child as a way to fulfill a healthy desire to live life more for themselves than ever before, or yes, even to stay young. Other women have lost children through accident or illness and want another baby, not to try to replace a loss that can never be restored but as a means of renewal and hope. Still other women in their forties who eye strollers or tiny layette outfits may feel a nameless longing for another child, a desire they can't fully describe.

When I talked with Maggie a couple of months after our first discussion, she said she was sleeping better. "The valerian helps, and I've been taking walks in the evenings by myself. I empty my mind for sleep." She also told me she was leaning against having another baby. She had weighed the impact of a third child on her ability to be an involved parent to her adolescent son and daughter, and on her career and finances. "I still have twinges of regret, but this feels like the best choice for me and the family," she said. Alison, however, still hopes to conceive a midlife baby. She's learned to respond to her protesting or disbelieving friends and relatives by saying, "Yes, I'll be a wiser, more experienced mother now than I was at twenty, and I'll have more fun too."

CHOICES TAKEN OUT OF OUR HANDS

Women who have struggled without success to conceive a baby often face critical and heart-rending decisions in their forties. The pain of infertility is frequently compounded by a lack of understanding on the part of others. The uninformed mistakenly assume that infertility is a plight of the spoiled and affluent, failing to recognize that it indiscriminately affects people of all ages, ethnicities, and economic statuses. Remarks from friends, family members, or co-workers are at best thoughtless and at worst cruel: "Aren't you pregnant yet? Well, you can always have fun trying." This remark was said by a co-worker with three children who had no inkling of how passionless and stressful making love becomes when it is part of a monthly cycle of hope and disappointment. Or: "There are enough children in the world anyway," a remark perhaps meant to comfort but that in truth only adds to the sting.

Then there is the jocular "I wish I had that problem. My three are driving me crazy—do you want them?" Or "Why don't you just adopt?" as if that decision were made easily and lightly.

The anguish of some women in their forties about infertility is made more acute because they are filled with doubt and grief about decisions they made earlier in their lives. Some women who had the option of having children in their twenties or thirties but elected not to now agonize over whether they did the right thing. They feel tortured, not knowing if they would have had the same trouble conceiving when they were younger or if they might have become pregnant more easily.

Women who got pregnant before but ended their pregnancy or gave up the child for adoption wonder whether their inability to conceive now is some form of retribution for that decision. Perhaps they had a child outside marriage, as a teenager. The stigma of shame and secrecy they experienced while young, unmarried, and pregnant haunts some of them continually; others, who buried their feelings about the pregnancy, birth, and adoption for years, now may find themselves face to face with these feelings. While certain religious faiths have programs especially to help women reconcile their feelings about having terminated a pregnancy in the past, less organized support exists for birth mothers whose children were adopted.

Some women who gave up a child for adoption seek contact with their child through adoption records. Others write letters or keep a journal, describing their feelings to the child they gave birth to but do not know, pouring out the rush of emotions, and setting out their hopes that the child's life is happy and secure. Women whose teenage pregnancy was a taboo family subject for decades sometimes confront that silence in their forties, bringing their stories out into the open and talking with parents and siblings about ways they may have been made to feel victimized and alone.

I have helped some of these women respond to unthinking comments about infertility by saying, "Infertility is a very serious and sensitive subject to me. I find your remarks difficult to listen to and upsetting." There is no simple way to assuage grief about childlessness, previous adoptions, or abortions, but making our way toward feeling mended can begin with a conscious acknowledgment of hurt and a clear goal of exchanging residual self-blame for forgiveness, and sorrow for peace.

INFERTILITY CAUSES AND EFFECTS

The reasons for female infertility in the forties vary. Women may no longer ovulate on a regular monthly schedule, which lowers our odds of conceiving. Some women conceive but miscarry very early, often before they have even missed their period. Jayne felt sure she was pregnant, although her period was only three days late. She had been trying to have a baby for nearly three years. She looked sorrowful as she described forcing herself to wait three days, then rushing to the drugstore for a home pregnancy test. "I got home and ran into the bathroom, but my period had started," she said. "I was crushed. I have a feeling I miscarried, because my period was so heavy and I had so much cramping that month. Besides, in all the years I've been trying to get pregnant, my period has never been three days late."

It's hard to know if Jayne indeed had a very early miscarriage. Some women have a condition called "late luteal phase defect," when their bodies do not produce enough progesterone during the second half of their menstrual cycle, the luteal phase. Because progesterone is vital in order to implant and sustain a fertilized egg successfully, its absence may be implicated in infertility. This may be particularly true as we age and our production of progesterone and other hormones declines.

I suggested that Jayne consider having her hormones measured to determine if low progesterone could be a variable in her inability to conceive. If her progesterone level was low, I explained that natural progesterone supplementation is benign and noninvasive and can be taken while a woman is trying to conceive. Some infertility specialists use progesterone supplementation during the first trimester of pregnancy to help sustain a fetus once a woman is pregnant. It turned out that Jayne's progesterone level was fine. She still wanted to conceive and intended to continue with her fertility specialist.

The older we get, the less viable for fertilization the eggs produced by our bodies may be. In some cases, no direct cause for the inability to conceive can be found. A woman in her forties who is dealing with infertility may decide that reproductive technology is appropriate and affordable. Others who try these highly sophisticated and very expensive methods to conceive may have to stop, either because they can't afford any more treatments or a certain number of attempts have failed. Gabrielle reached that point after her second attempt at in-vitro fertilization using donor eggs was unsuccessful. She was 42, and the fertility specialist she and her husband were working with said there was no clinical reason not to try a third time if they wanted to. But after many tears, she and her husband decided not to go through the cycle again, which taxed them physically, emotionally, and financially.

"We could have kept going, because there's always the hope that conception and full-term pregnancy will happen next time," said Gabrielle. "But we had to look at what it would do to both of us if we had another unsuccessful attempt. Also, the third attempt would have depleted our financial reserves completely. I'm glad we went as far as we did to have a biological child," she continued, "because at first I wasn't going to have any treatment. I didn't think I could take the stress. But I found strength I didn't know I had."

The escalations of hope followed by the sharp descents into disappointment had placed a great strain on her marriage, Gabrielle said. "I thought I was going to end up without a husband too. We've weathered the shakiest times. We've come through the experience of infertility with the realization that we are committed to this marriage, with or without children."

For some women who want to build a family, adoption is a viable option, but if they are married to men who prefer to remain childless rather than adopt, these differing goals are not simple to resolve. Beth said, "I know my husband and I could be loving parents. I think our purpose in that role is larger than replicating our DNA, but my husband feels strongly about having biological children. We went through a period where neither of us was listening to the other about this issue. I thought he was being completely egotistical and selfish, and he saw my feelings as a highly romanticized view of what it would really be like to adopt a child."

Beth is 41 and her husband is 44. Finally they sought help from a counselor, who guided them to a point where they were going to explore adoption step by step, making a decision at each point. "This approach really works for me," Beth said. "We're not saying we're going to go full steam ahead and adopt, but we're not ruling it out either. We've both agreed that our overarching goal is to be a loving family, whether that's two of us or eventually more. With that goal in mind, we can evaluate all of our options. If any part of the adoption process feels like too much of a threat to our family stability, we'll reassess."

CHOICES OTHERS HAVE MADE

Mary reconciled herself, not without struggle, to the fact that when she married her fiancé, whom she had known for five years, they would not have children. "He was very clear right from the beginning that he didn't want children," Mary said. She was in her late thirties when she began this relationship; now 42, she acknowledged that she might not have considered the full implications of her fiancé's choice when they first discussed the issue. "Maybe I thought he would change his mind, or maybe the issue of children seemed less important in our giddy early days together. About two years ago I went through what could be called a crisis about the issue. I was pressuring him about having children, saying things like 'I know you didn't want children before, but I thought you would want them with *me*.' He reminded me that he had laid out his feelings very clearly and had never given me any impression that it would be otherwise. I thought I had accepted it, but on some level I guess I hadn't."

Mary contemplated ending her relationship with him and in fact she stopped seeing him for a time. At the time, they hadn't yet agreed to marry. "I thought I'd start over, but the fact was, I missed him terribly, and I don't think there is anyone more suitable for me out there. I could go looking, and maybe I would meet someone who is willing to have children later in life. But that person wouldn't have all the qualities that made me fall in love with him."

Mary and her fiancé eventually healed their rift and were set to marry at the end of the year. Even though she decided to accept life without children, she didn't entirely get over her sense that that wasn't exactly what she had planned. "I still want to be important in a child's life," she told me. "I have two nephews I've decided to see more often. My neighbor across the street is a single mother with two small kids. They've been running out to greet me lately, especially since they've started to see me walking. Even though it looks like my own children aren't going to be part of the grand scheme of my life, I still want to make time to create a role for myself as a mentor and friend to children I care about."

PREVENTING PREGNANCY IN THE FORTIES

Women in their forties have a high rate of unplanned pregnancies. In some cases a midlife baby comes along because a woman mistakenly assumes she is no longer fertile and stops using birth control prematurely. Or a woman who has previously been successful at charting her fertile periods and using birth control during those times learns, through an unanticipated pregnancy, that she can no longer accurately predict when she is ovulating because her cycle is now irregular.

"I was a 'change of life' baby myself," says Linda, 40. "My mother was forty-two when she had me, and I know I wasn't planned. My oldest brother is going to be 60. I'm just getting to the point where my own children are a little more independent now that they're eleven and thirteen. They still need plenty of supervision, but as long as I know where they are and whom they're with now, I can be comfortable letting them plan something for a weekend afternoon. I want to be sure I don't have a surprise baby like my mother did."

We may look at our birth control options differently in our forties than we did when we were younger. Many forties women tell me they would like to switch their form of birth control but don't know of another option that suits their lifestyle. Others ask if they can stop using it altogether, to which I always respond, "Only if an unplanned pregnancy would be acceptable."

Some health care practitioners prescribe low-dose oral contraceptives, with their combination of estrogen and synthetic progestin, to manage perimenopausal symptoms. These low-dose birth control pills may be a good option for women who find that they relieve their hot flashes or night sweats and who also do not wish to become pregnant. For them, a birth control choice serves the dual purpose of providing perimenopausal symptom relief as well. But for many women the synthetic hormones in oral contraceptives have unpleasant side effects, such as weight gain, mood changes, and insomnia. For these women, birth control choices can be difficult. A barrier form of birth control, such as a condom and/or diaphragm, is probably the best choice, short of a vasectomy for their partner.

The forties may also be a time when our attitudes about birth control change. Some women in their forties tell me they're tired of taking full responsibility for birth control and wish their husbands would use condoms or have a vasectomy. But old habits die hard, and they're not sure how to broach this subject. I usually recommend framing this conversation in terms of shared responsibility, an approach Tammy found useful. She had been using a diaphragm for years, but in recent months she found it more annoying and messy than she had in the past. She also thought the diaphragm might be partly responsible for the bladder infections she had had this year. It's true that a diaphragm is sometimes linked to an inflammation or infection that affects the bladder, and during our forties, when vaginal tissue becomes more susceptible to infection, this can happen more often.

"When you talk about this with your husband, rather than focus on the fact that you're tired of using the diaphragm, talk first about how you love being close with him," I recommended to Tammy. "Then you can turn the discussion toward your desire that your husband share the responsibility for birth control by letting him know you'd like a feeling of freedom and spontaneity occasionally too."

Neither Tammy nor her husband were ready to go for surgical sterilization through tubal ligation or vasectomy, but they did reach a compromise where they would alternate between using a condom and a diaphragm. "We decided to try it month by month and see what happens. We thought it would be tedious to try to keep track of whose week it was, so we'll try the thirty-day plan.

"My husband wasn't thrilled at first, but I told him this was important to me. We ended up making a deal as a kind of joke to break the tension," Tammy said. "I told him that during the months when he had to be in charge of buying and using birth control, and I didn't have to bother with the diaphragm, I'd probably feel like making love twice as often. He liked that idea." Tammy is accustomed to using spermicide with her diaphragm, but I suggested that her husband look for condoms with spermicide in the tip for more protection, since they don't want to have more children.

It's important for women in their forties who do not want to become pregnant to have adequate birth control, even if their menstrual cycle has become irregular. We have a lot going on in our forties — physical and emotional changes, family milestones, career crossroads. If an unplanned pregnancy would be okay with you, you can be sporadic about birth control. But if a pregnancy would add an element of uncertainty or even risk into an already complex decade, be sure that intercourse is protected.

DUELING MOOD SWINGS

A perimenopausal woman who has teenagers in the house undergoing their own adolescent hormonal changes can feel like, on any given day, the family mood swings are all over the map. "There are times when I could honestly believe our family belongs in a tabloid because we've all been abducted by aliens and some other creatures are inhabiting our bodies," said Tina. "My two sweet sons have become so selfish and sullen. And I come home from work on many days feeling like I want to start crying or yelling or both."

The collision of teenage changes and the perimenopausal transition is enough to make us think the gods are playing a joke on us, and not a very funny one at that. I asked Tina what would happen if she and her teenage sons sat down so she could explain some of what she is going through. She grew thoughtful for a moment and said, "Yes, I could do that." I told her that this conversation could be an opportunity for her to make a very valuable connection with her sons, by trusting them enough to let them know what might be happening with her hormones and how they could seem to play tricks on her body and emotions. She might even want to compare her own situation with the hormonal fluctuations her sons were going through.

Children can readily understand the concept of something in your body being out of balance, but it's important to impress upon children that you aren't ill. "You can tell your boys that the imbalance is something that can be restored, and describe what you're doing to help that by eating differently and taking black cohosh. You can also explain that when your hormones, which are chemicals, are changing, there can be physical and emotional effects, like fatigue and irritability."

I also suggested that Tina give her sons a role in helping her if possible. "You could ask one or both of them to take a walk with you, explaining that exercise helps keep your body in balance. If they're at that stage where being seen in public with Mom embarrasses them, tell them you want an hour of peace and quiet every evening. Let them pick the hour, but make sure they understand that they aren't to be fighting, playing the stereo or television, or interrupting you. Let them know that the time for you to unwind is very important for your health."

Tina wasn't so sure how it would be to talk with her sons about these issues. Like many mothers who focus their energy and time more on what the family needs than on their own needs, she wasn't used to the idea of asking her children for anything. "But they're thirteen and fifteen now," I pointed out. "That's a perfect time to give them more responsibility for the health of the family."

"I was really proud of them," Tina told me, when I asked her a few weeks later how the conversation with her sons had gone. "They seemed embarrassed at first when I started to explain that my hormones are changing. Maybe they thought I was going to say something really personal. But they both have deep voices now, so I just said they had each experienced something similar when hormones had changed their voices. My youngest son asked me if I was sick—you were right to remind me to be sure they understand that I'm not," she said.

"They actually listened when I told them I was trying to eat differently and exercise to make my body feel more in balance, and that I was taking an herb. My youngest son was quite interested. He's in an advanced science class and wanted to know if we could grow our own crop of black cohosh."

The quiet hour in the evenings was also good for the whole family, Tina reported. "I can't tell you how many times I would come home from work and yell about the noise, or the clothes on the floor, or a noisy argument they were having. But when I told them that it was important for my health that evenings not be chaos, it seemed like it made a different impression on them, not just Mom nagging again.

"Oh, I won't say they suddenly started being quiet in the evening for an hour," Tina continued. "They had trouble deciding at first what hour it would be and had to fight about that for a while, but I just let them work it out. Then my fifteen-year-old was calling it 'lockdown,' like in a prison rebellion, but I didn't react. I just told them that I really appreciated that they were willing to make some changes that would be helpful to me."

Then her sons started to use the quiet hour to get most of their homework done, which pleased Tina. "I don't have to ask seven times if their homework is done. And I don't have to compete with the television because we've agreed that it's off during this hour. Sometimes the hour is up and they still are reading or studying, and no one turns on the TV for the rest of the evening," she said.

The effects of Tina's explanation and request to her sons actually reverberated throughout the family, which surprised her. "Now I can come home knowing that at some point during the evening I get to relax. It's made a big difference in the way I feel."

"It's amazing what a discussion about balance and wholeness can do for the whole family," I said.

NEW RITES AND RITUALS

It's not only teenagers at home, like Tina's sons, who test our composure when we're experiencing perimenopausal mood changes. Older children who challenge long-standing rules or criticize family traditions can make us feel rejected, depressed, defensive, or all three, and these emotions may collide with perimenopausal mood changes that are hormonally driven. "Suddenly everything I put on the table is up for judgment and then refusal by my twenty-one-year-old daughter," said Carol, 46. "Food I've served for years now causes pollution or world hunger. I've snapped at her that I'm not running a restaurant, and she almost never eats with us anymore. I miss the family time we used to have when we were together at meals."

"Could you have her shop for and prepare some of your meals?" I asked Carol. Carol had begun to eat more phytoestrogenic foods, but she wasn't familiar with cooking with soy protein like tofu, tempeh, and miso. "Your daughter might enjoy cooking a vegetarian meal, it would defuse the arguments about what you serve, and it would give you a break, all at the same time," I suggested.

Carol and I also talked about her missing the family time around the dinner table. "Even though I've always worked full time, I've made sure we were together at dinner time," she said. "But now that the kids are older, it seems like they're scattered here and there. The boys have practice for one sport or another depending on the season, and if my daughter has an evening class, she doesn't come home for dinner."

"Your children probably want to exercise some independence now that they're older and have lots of interests outside the home. Maybe you can change the dinner routine so you don't feel as frustrated when the children aren't there. Your daughter may not be as critical of your cooking as she sounds. It could be part of an inarticulate wish that she were living independently like some of her friends."

"Yes, she wanted very badly to live in an apartment this year, but my husband and I couldn't swing an apartment and tuition and books too. We gave her the choice: continue her education with our help, but that meant living at home; or get a job and an apartment like a lot of her friends. She really wanted to finish her degree," Carol explained.

I suggested that Carol find one or two evenings a week when her husband and children could be together for the mealtime that she considered an important family tradition. "Agreeing on one or two nights a week might be easier than trying to coordinate schedules every night," I said. "Your daughter and your sons can take turns being the chef. It changes the routine, yet you don't have to let go of having your husband and children with you for meals."

"Well, we're writing a cookbook," Carol announced on the phone when we spoke two months later. "My daughter has perfected a wonderful pasta sauce with tofu in it, my oldest son makes a great pizza, and the younger one seems to have a flair for dessert." Carol said that Wednesday and Sunday evenings are a new family tradition with her visiting chefs. "We've had a few missteps," she said. "My daughter made something with garbanzo beans and curry that was the most amazing fluorescent yellow color and had the oddest taste and a pasty consistency. Everyone was very game at first, trying to eat it and not say anything, which I thought was very respectful. But then my thirteen-year-old couldn't help himself and started snickering when he raised a big lump of it up on his fork and it stayed there, completely immobile. That was it. We all shrieked with laughter. My daughter acted huffy for a few minutes, but then even she had to laugh because our dog wouldn't go near it when we put some in his dish. My sons called it Garbanzo Epoxy. We'll probably laugh about that for the next thirty years, especially when we think of the few moments when we all tried to chew it."

Many women I know who are in their forties create all kinds of new rituals for themselves, to relax, to write down their feelings, to move their bodies, to awaken their senses. We can use the same creativity to create new rituals and traditions with our families, to breathe new life into things we've done for years. It doesn't have to be hurtful that a tradition seems to be unraveling—it can be our opportunity to involve the family in a new interest or rite. Carol involved her family in her experiment with new foods, and she planned to have each of her three children bring one of their special dishes to the next holiday gathering at her husband's parents' home. "All three kids have grumbled about going for the last couple of years. They say it's boring. I think they'll take more of an interest if they get a chance to show off their cooking for all the relatives," she said.

As our children get older and test their independence, they can act in ways that embarrass and stress us. Janice got a call at two A.M. one morning from the police—her 18-year-old stepson had been taken into custody when police broke up a large outdoor party where minors were drinking, after neighbors complained about the noise. "I was awake," Janice said. "Actually I was thinking about my mother because I had talked to her on the phone that evening and she sounded very vague." Janice's mother had been showing signs of forgetfulness, which was a big concern since she lived three hundred miles away. "Jason told us he was staying at his friend Ryan's house, which he sometimes does. I know Ryan's parents, so I didn't think anything was unusual. But evidently Ryan's parents were gone for the weekend, and a hundred kids showed up at the house for a big blowout of a party."

Janice folded her hands in her lap. "I think I aged fifty years when the police officer identified himself on the phone. In the few seconds before he told me Jason was cited for underage drinking and drinking in public and that we needed to come and get him, I thought all kinds of horrible things — car accident, hospital, you name it." Her voice quavered slightly.

"My husband has joint custody of Jason with his ex-wife. She has two children with her current husband and I swear it seems like she's written Jason off and assumed that because my husband and I didn't have children together, we can take care of all of Jason's needs. I've been his stepmother since he was six years old, and although we've had our ups and downs, I'm very attached to him. I'm so disappointed, I can hardly speak to him, and I'm very worried besides. How much is he drinking? I'm sure this wasn't a single incident, and I have no way to monitor what he does when he's at his mother's. Do I have to start calling his friends' parents now every time he's spending time with them? I thought we had established much more trust than that."

"Disappointment and trust are powerful words — you used both of them just now," I said. "Did you say those things to Jason?" Janice took off her glasses and rubbed her eyes before she answered. "No, actually we said that we were very angry. We told him there were consequences of his behavior and that he can't see his friends for the next month, or at least the portion of the month that he's with us."

When Janice first visited my office, she had been very concerned about a few episodes of forgetfulness on the job; she had resolved that problem by turning over more responsibility to her assistant. I suggested that she borrow her work technique of turning over some responsibility to help deal with this incident with her stepson.

"You can explain very directly, just as you did to me, that your trust in him has been very badly damaged, and that you're deeply disappointed," I said. "If you think you can, you might leave it up to him to determine how he's going to reestablish your trust. Tell him that you want him to figure that out, and let you know what he intends to do to earn back the trust he's lost."

"I like the sound of that," Janice said. "Because that really is true. We can ground him for a month, but after the month is up, there's no way to know if anything is different unless he's made some kind of commitment we can see that the behavior won't continue."

Because Janice and I are in regular contact as we continue to work on her insomnia and rising stress level, we spoke about her stepson again the following week. "Talking about being so let down was very effective," Janice said. "He looked crushed, as opposed to just kind of defiant, the way he was the day after we got the call from the police and my husband and I were still so angry. Jason didn't seem to know how to answer when I told him we were leaving it up to him to earn back our faith in him, and that we still had enough trust in him to think he could develop a plan to do that. At first I thought, 'Uh-oh, this is going to backfire — he's going to tell us he doesn't care that we don't trust him anymore.'"

I heard Janice take a deep breath on the other end of the phone. "But he actually asked what I thought was a wise question. He wanted to know if we thought he could also earn his mother and stepfather's trust again, as well as Ryan's parents', who were also bitterly disappointed that the police had been summoned to their house while they were away. We told him we thought he probably could. Then he talked about not sneaking around and planning parties at homes where there are no adults, and being honest about what he's doing. The drinking was a tougher part of the discussion. He seemed to think that agreeing not to drink and drive was enough, but we held firm. We told him that for the two and a half years until it's legal for him to drink alcohol, we didn't want him to drink at our house, his friends' houses, or anywhere else. We stayed on the message of legality, and maturity, which means respecting certain regulations."

Maybe it's wishful thinking or a false sense of nostalgia for a supposedly easier time, but it does seem that raising children now is much more complicated and expensive than it was when we were growing up. Nancy, whose two children were in college, talked about the financial pressure of trying to help put two students through school at once. "We've saved for their education since both of them were born, but not enough to meet the expenses of two private schools. They both will be repaying loans after they finish, and my husband and I work a lot of overtime. Our kids grew much faster than our savings plan, unfortunately." Nancy also had concerns because it looked like she and her husband, who were both 48, wouldn't be able to retire for another twenty-five years since they were still allocating large sums of money for their children's education. "I didn't finish college so it does make me feel very good that I'm in a position to help my children. They're both doing so well in school," Nancy said.

"Would you ever consider finishing school yourself now?" I asked Nancy. "I'd probably have to start all over, and it might take ten years," she said. "Those ten years will fly by anyway, whether you decide to go back to school or not," I said. I raised this issue with Nancy for two reasons: I happened to know that her employer had a tuition assistance program for employees who were pursuing studies related to their jobs, so I thought it was worthwhile that she look into that program. Also, because she had voiced her concern about working lots of overtime and possibly being very far from retirement, it occurred to me that additional education and training might help her advance professionally.

"It also just might feel great to finish something you started thirty years ago," I said. Nancy decided to enroll in a special program for working adults with night and weekend classes, although she was anxious about returning to school after many years. "It's been so long since I've studied, and I don't know if I'll have enough time to keep up with classes and my job."

"I love it," she said enthusiastically when I asked her how her classes were going a month after she started. "It's hard to force myself to concentrate and study, but I'm getting better at it. I'm learning a lot, but I also find that all my years of work experience are useful in some of my classes too. It's wonderful to be working toward this goal for myself at the same time I'm helping my children to achieve something important. My children are excited and proud of me. They promised to give me some hints on getting ready for exams."

TIPPING THE SCALE

Women who work outside the home and who have children who still need supervision are often torn between untenable choices. Skip an important soccer match, or face a supervisor's disapproval for leaving work early. Send a sick child to the babysitter's, or stay home and miss a key deadline. The decade of the forties can also bring the confluence of multiple rigorous demands: critical points along their career path, and children reaching adolescence, often needing more guidance and direction than they did as grade-schoolers. Just the logistics of keeping children's lives and schedules organized can be daunting today. Our world is less safe, so many children don't have the luxury of running free in their neighborhood to play with other children. Play dates have to be scheduled, verified, and kept. Children are also involved in many more activities than they were a generation ago, requiring a detailed transportation schedule to get them to and from practice, lessons, and appointments.

Add perimenopausal memory changes into this mix, and you have all the ingredients for confusion, guilt, and overload. "I consider myself a detail person, the one who keeps lists and gets things done. Now I feel like I've gone soft in the head. I notice that my children are saying 'Mom, I *told* you already' to me a lot, but I could swear I'm hearing these things for the first time," said Pat. "How much of it is their last-minute demands, and how much of it is my being distracted or forgetful, I don't know. I'm ready to install a videocamera in our house so I can play back all the conversations."

Pat's facetious threat had a valid ring to it—she did need help keeping rides, pickup times, permission slips, and practice schedules straight for her children, 12-year-old twins and a 10-year-old. "You don't have to communicate the details of your shifting hormone levels, mood swings, or memory changes," I said, "but you can let your children know what's going on by telling them you have a big list of things to do and that you need help."

I suggested that Pat and her husband sit down with their three children once a week to review who would be going where and to coordinate schedules. This would accomplish two key goals. First, she and her husband could divide up more of the responsibility for making sure their children were where they needed to be. Second, it would give the family an opportunity to prioritize their activities each week and decide if anything could be let go. Pat was very proud of her children's involvement in sports and other after-school activities, but she conceded that keeping their appointments sometimes interfered with her work and made her feel that she was being run ragged. "You don't have to say yes to everything," I reminded Pat. "It's acceptable to let your children know that you need time to focus on your work. They can also understand that you would like some downtime when everyone is home.

"All politicians have schedulers who handle their calendars. Maybe your twins could take this role and keep a master calendar after each family meeting. You can decide when you want 'Mom's time out,' and that gets put on the schedule too, just like play rehearsals and ballet lessons," I said.

Before she instituted the family calendar, Pat had kept her own schedule organized as well as her children's. She often felt frazzled and overloaded as she looked at the day's schedule, with too little time between appointments and commitments. Giving the whole family a share of the responsibility worked out well for her. "My twins pointed out that there was no way I could get from point A to point B on time when we discussed the upcoming week, so we figured out a different plan. It was great," she said.

A very straightforward and honest request for help can actually help build family harmony and support for you and your efforts to take optimum care of yourself during your forties. You're also acting as a role model by demonstrating that your health and well-being are important. I've often suggested that women adopt the same strategy with their employers when shifting family demands come into play. Jacqueline's work day ended at 5:30; her two junior high school daughters finished school at 3:35. They took part in supervised after-school activities two, sometimes three days a week, but there were at least two days when Jacqueline worried about where they were and what they were doing until she arrived home shortly before six.

"Talk to your employer about flexibility two afternoons a week," I suggested to Jacqueline. "If you present your case in terms of balancing your commitment to your job along with your need to supervise your teenage daughters, you may be able to work something out. If you worked until four o'clock twice a week, you could take work home and be available by phone for that last hour. Stress your absolute commitment to getting the work done, and offer to test a flexible schedule for thirty days. That way you negotiate from a position of strength."

Jacqueline's conversation with her employer was very successful. "He agreed to try the flexible schedule and told me he valued me as an employee and appreciated my work. He said he knew I wouldn't be asking for this flexibility if it wasn't important. I wasn't sure how he was going to react to my request, but I felt like I had been listened to and respected," Jacqueline said.

Listened to and respected—the response we can expect when we know our own priorities, identify what we require for our mental and physical health, and make those needs clear to family, friends, and co-workers in our circle.

REBUILDING THE NEST

For women in their forties, children leaving home is also a time of mixed emotions. On one hand we may have trouble believing they're really old enough to be capable of being on their own—how can they not need us anymore? We may think back with poignancy to when they were small, helpless, and utterly dependent on us. One woman I know used a supermarket analogy. "When my babies were out of diapers, I'd walk down the aisle and say, 'I don't need those anymore.' Then I walked down the aisle with the sanitary supplies and Midol, and I realized that my daughters needed that but I wouldn't for much longer, and soon they'd leave home and I wouldn't buy these things for them anymore. What aisle do I head for next?"

Leaving home is a major milestone in the series of steps children take toward independence, each one poignant in its own way. I remember my husband's puzzlement when I tearfully told him our oldest son, then six, had lost his first perfect little baby tooth. "Well, isn't that supposed to happen?" he asked cautiously. "But you don't understand," I remember saying, almost in anguish. "He's not a baby anymore."

When young men and women who were babies only the blink of an eye ago leave home, we inherit a cavernous feeling somewhere in our hearts, even if we do look forward to the additional freedom. If your children are going out into the world, I suggest you have your own graduation of sorts to mark this significant time in your career as a mother:

- ✦ Start by acknowledging the feelings you have about this change in your life, whether it is a sense of loss or relief, or a mixture of both. Whether they strike out for a college across the country or for the next town to live in an apartment, it's still a big change not to see your children daily, and you can expect to miss them, even if your relationship with them has been stormy at times.

- ✦ Review your strengths as a parent. Think about the qualities, knowledge, and traditions your children are taking out into the world that you gave them. Much of what they will become will reflect your importance in their life.

- ✦ Take time to consider the ways you want to continue to act as your children's mentor after they leave home.

- ✦ Talk to other women whose children have left home, and take comfort in hearing about what it was like for them. When my oldest son was getting ready to leave home for the first time, my dear friend Nancy provided me with such solace. Her oldest was already out in the world, and she gently reminded me that children do come back, for holidays, for advice, for companionship on different terms. "A child leaving home isn't an event but a process," she said, sensible words that sustained me through a time of strong and mixed emotions.

- ✦ Have a discussion with your spouse about this change in your lives. He may share some of your feelings about seeing a child become an adult, and recollections about all you've both learned through parenthood can be mutually reassuring.

◆ Most important, decide on what you would like to gain from this change in your life: more solitude for yourself, additional time with your spouse, a different dynamic with the child who has left home, or a change in your relationship with other children who are still at home are all possibilities.

REFEATHERING OUR NESTS

When we are in our forties, parents or other older relatives can become more a part of our nests, sometimes presenting difficult choices and stretching our reserves of strength, time, and even financial resources.

Janice had been worried about her mother for some months, fearing that she was developing Alzheimer's disease when she would sound vague or forgetful on the phone. She made a trip to visit her mother three hundred miles away and came back troubled about what might lie ahead.

"Mother is definitely undergoing some changes," she told me. "I wouldn't say she has senile dementia, but she didn't seem to be as on top of things as she once was. The place was a mess with bills and papers everywhere, and I didn't know what needed attention or which bills had to be paid. My mother has always been very independent so it wasn't appropriate that I ask or start going through things. The house has become too much for her—it's too big and falling into disrepair. Either she doesn't notice, or she doesn't want to spend the money now. I don't know what to do. I've thought about moving her in with us."

The timing of Janice's visit to her mother coincided with the stress of her stepson's surreptitious partying and the middle-of-the-night phone call that every parent dreads. Several months earlier, when she first saw me for her perimenopausal symptoms, we had focused on improving her memory and concentration and alleviating her insomnia and hot flashes. She decided to try an herbal approach, using ginkgo biloba to improve her concentration and black cohosh to help with hot flashes and insomnia. Her symptoms had almost disappeared, but the high stress she was experiencing about her mother and stepson seemed to cause a setback, particularly with her insomnia. Since returning from the visit to her mother's, she said she had slept poorly for a week and felt muddled and distracted during the day.

Janice seemed very distraught as we talked, so I reminded her how crucial it was that she take care of herself. "If your stepson is going to need more supervision and you have your mother's situation in front of you at the same time, you'll need to be strong and rested," I said.

"You won't be able to figure out all the steps involved in your mother's care in one day, so let's think about the sequence," I suggested. I thought Janice should start by getting a copy of the yellow pages from her mother's community—she had a high school friend there whom she could ask to send her one—to begin to identify resources she might need, such as local health care providers, geriatric social workers, assisted living possibilities, and adult day care. "I know it's very hard to witness your mother's changes," I said. "But as long as you feel she's not in danger now, you can start to put a plan in place to meet each need as it arises. You don't necessarily have to move her in with you—that might not be best for her or you."

Janice nodded.

"Look at all the problem solving you've done during the last several months," I said, reminding her that she was managing her symptoms of perimenopause and making changes in her work. "The same approach will work where your mother is concerned." Janice seemed relieved that she didn't have to rush to assume all responsibility for her mother yet. I suggested that she use her valuable organizational skills to devise the best plan to let her mother maintain as much control of her life as possible, and to give herself the sense that she was being proactive. "If your mother does need more serious intervention later, you'll be that much more prepared," I said.

Babies, adolescents, college students, and older relatives in our nests—the job is never simple, or easy. We can do our very best, although at times that may not be enough to protect the people we love against the occasional indifferent turn of events. But there are certainties we bring to relationships that span the generations: the wisdom that says our health is a primary concern no matter how taxing the demands of the family may be, the maturity to distinguish between generous giving of ourselves and self-sacrifice that actually harms us, and the confidence that comes with knowing that it is our energy and love that suffuse the family with spirit.

SHARING YOUR HISTORY

In the course of writing this book, I met with a discussion group of women to whom I am eternally grateful. My purpose was to ensure that when I finished this project, no one would approach me and say, "I really wish you had discussed — — — or presented — — —." What came out of those evenings were several wonderful ideas, one of which I want to offer here.

The suggestion was that I offer women ways to chronicle our personal history, so that we can pass along stories about the changes we experience in our forties to our children or others. These women commented, "If only I had more information about what my mother experienced in her forties, I might have more of an idea of what to expect." Other women saw developing a personal history as a meaningful exercise to explore more about themselves, a way of taking a journey into themselves.

Scan the shelves in any bookstore, and you'll find a host of guides to help you write an autobiography or compile a family history. These books include sections on writing family trees, holiday traditions, the price of gas and other goods, favorite recipes, and gardening secrets.

Sharing recollections and putting together family lore is a rich and deeply feminine tradition, assuring that women's wisdom has continuity through the years. Writing the history of your forties may help you clarify some of your experiences, and if you choose, it can become a gift for your children or for other family members. During the discussion group, each of us recognized that writing accounts of our own struggles, experiences, and triumphs might help smooth the path for those who would follow us.

When I considered including a section on writing a personal history in this book, I realized that it might seem overwhelming to some women—one more thing to do on an already too-long list. That's why I'm suggesting that the process be guided. In other words, it's not the same as sitting down with empty pages and proceeding to write your story (even though, if you are so inclined, that would be wonderful). Maybe some of you have already begun to write a family history and will add the details about this transitional decade to that story. I am going to try to guide you gently through some questions that may illuminate certain points for you and help you create a picture of your experiences. I don't see us writing martyrs' tales but stories about courage, strength, and perseverance during a time when we had no map to follow.

Maybe you're thinking, "But I don't like to write," or "I'm not good at it." Your writing style, punctuation, and grammar are less important than simply telling your story in your own way, whether you intend to share it with others or are writing to enlighten yourself. Believe me, if you have children, they'll truly appreciate one day that this is "vintage Mom." The main suggestion I have is that you create no expectations for yourself, so that whatever develops can do so naturally and spontaneously. When you're ready to start writing your history, you may find that carrying around a small notebook is helpful, allowing you to record anything that comes to mind. I find that when I'm involved in a writing project, ideas come at the craziest times, such as when I'm waiting in line at the grocery store or stopped in traffic. If I have something to write on, I can capture the thought and record it later where it needs to be.

You may find that as you go through this exercise, you will want to write more in response to certain questions than others. Even that will be a revealing indication about subjects where you are comfortable and those where you have more questions about yourself.

To make this history as personal as possible, I strongly suggest that you include your experiences, impressions, and concerns about your friends, family, or children whenever it seems appropriate. If you decide to pass this personal history on, whoever reads it will treasure the fact that you have taken the time to write your story for them and will be touched as they read about their part in your life.

In the course of your lifetime as a baby boomer, you have seen amazing changes in the field of women's health. Speaking for myself, I have gone from having children when Lamaze was just being intro-

duced in Milwaukee, to the present, when many health care practitioners won't deliver a baby unless the mother has participated in childbirth
education classes. Think about that—we have been privileged to be a
part of reclaiming our bodies. We have gone from our mothers' "knock
out, drag out" childbirths to becoming very active participants in everything that concerns our health: in giving birth, caring for our bodies, and
identifying which foods, vitamins, and exercises are right for us and our
families. We no longer accept being patronized or patted on the shoul-
der but assume full responsibility for our share of the partnership with
our health care provider. Now that we're in our forties, we're recasting
the molds again, changing the way this decade is viewed and asking for
full attention from the medical community. Write about the distinctive
rhythm of your journey in as much detail as you can.

If, after finishing your history, you decide that it reveals too much
about you, you can always edit what you have written, keep the original
copy for yourself, and give a revised edition to whomever you wish.
Many of us find the process of writing therapeutic and discover that the
simple act of putting something on paper brings clarity and balance
where there was once confusion or distress. Thinking about and
responding to the questions at the end of this chapter may be a great tool
to help you work through issues that are important to you right now. Or
writing your story may also direct you back to past health care issues that
remain unresolved.

Keep in mind that you can complete your story at your own pace
and in any format you like. You can keep your story in a separate notebook or on your home computer. You may go back to fill in portions of
this history over several weeks, months, or even years. The main goal is
for you to have a story that will shed light on what this journey was like
for you. My wish for you is that you enjoy creating this part of your
legacy, and that you learn more about yourself as you do.

GETTING STARTED

Before you start writing your personal history, take a few moments to
find a quiet place that has the feeling of a sanctuary for you. Turn off the

noise of daily life, and shift into a more contemplative state, trying this brief interlude of relaxation:

> Position yourself comfortably and close your eyes. For two to five minutes, focus only on breathing out and breathing in. You may need to make several attempts before this simple exercise brings you to a more calm and centered frame of mind, but keep practicing. The very act of stopping for a few minutes and making a conscious effort to be slow, quiet, and peaceful is a very healthy practice. You may decide to do it each time you start to write parts of your story.

FINDING YOUR VOICE

The details that seem most vivid to you are what will bring your story to life — what you felt like when you first realized your body was changing, what it is like if your emotions threaten to get out of control, your thoughts about what really matters at this time in your life, and what prompted you to seek help if you have done so. Some women have told me about physical cues that alerted them to their body's changes: a hot flash in the middle of a business meeting or an episode of very uncomfortable lovemaking. For other women, it was mental or emotional signals that made them realize that things were different: forgetting to pick up a child from softball practice or breaking down in angry tears at a family gathering. Many forties women talk to me about changes that cause them to take stock of their purpose, to question what they were doing and why, and to seek renewed and deeper meaning in all aspects of their lives.

You may also find it helpful to ask yourself what you would have liked your mother to convey or share if she had kept a journal about *her* perimenopause. Three women I've talked with reflected on this question:

Annette _____

My mother was unaware that she was going through perimenopause in her forties. If she had been clear that there was such a thing, then maybe she would have had something helpful to share with me. The way I see it, she had no knowledge that there was anything called perimenopause or that anybody experienced symptoms. I remember it seemed to me that my parents' relationship changed during that time and that they had a lot of problems. I guess now that I'm in my forties, I'm curious to know how their relationship suffered because of her perimenopausal symptoms. I wonder what portion of their problems as a couple could have been alleviated if someone had been able to identify the changes with and for her. Perhaps if she could have known that what she felt was more than just middle age, their marriage would have gone more smoothly in those years. She was not able to communicate to my dad what was happening. I think if she had been, my dad would have been more supportive.

Belinda

I would have liked for my mother just to tell me what her forties were like for her. I'd like to know if perimenopausal symptoms are hereditary, and if I can expect to go through similar physical and emotional changes. I have no idea if she even went through perimenopausal symptoms before she stopped menstruating completely, and if she did, how it was. I read once in her diary that she suffered from depression. I would love to know if it was related to perimenopause. I also remember her being away for a while — my grandmother told me she was in an institution. When she came back, she never told me where she had been, why she went away, or what treatment she had. I wonder if they even talked about perimenopause back then, or if she was simply considered psychologically ill.

Charlene

I would love to know from my mother, first of all, if she experienced perimenopause. If she did, how old was she? What were some of her symptoms? Who or what helped her? How did it affect the way she felt about us kids, and about our dad?

MY GRANDMOTHER'S STORY

Shortly after Charlene, Annette, Belinda, and the other women in the discussion group talked about the value of a personal history, I decided to get out the journals that my grandmother, Inez Hiar Forman, kept all her life. I reread the entries she made in the 1920s and 1930s, when she was in her forties. She wrote in leather-bound books, some large, some smaller, with different-colored covers, from the time she married in her teens until shortly before she died at age 86. These hundreds of pages in her lovely handwriting describe everything about her life: what the crops were like in a given season on her Michigan farm, how many pickles she canned, when she was unhappy with family members, who came to visit, whose birthday was being celebrated, and whose death was being mourned.

My grandmother's journals are a family treasure. She called them her "Bibles," and to this day, we pull them out to settle any family argument about what actually happened — it's all there in remarkable detail. I can read about the day my parents were married, the day I was born, and the day she became a great-grandmother when I had my first son.

In rereading what she wrote in her forties, some of what I found seems to clearly reflect that she was in her perimenopausal transition. Of course, that transition remained unrecognized and unnamed for six more decades and is still only gradually being acknowledged as a legitimate passage in a woman's life. Some might argue that I'm reading too much into what my grandmother wrote. But I don't think it's a coincidence that her entries during that time seem more focused on herself and the changes she experienced, although she may not have fully understood them.

My grandmother's life on the farm may seem a world away from our modern experience, untethered as she was to phone, fax, e-mail or laptop, unconcerned as she was about crime in her tranquil setting. But her words echo in many ways my own personal experience in my forties, and much of what countless women have described to me.

Here is what my grandmother wrote about her changing moods:

March 15, 1929, age 46:
"The weather has been blustery and so have I."

April 2, 1925, age 42:
"Nasty, rainy weather, just like my mood."

December 14, 1930, age 48:
"I'm so tearful."

About sleep disturbances:

December 29, 1930, age 48:
"If I could just get a good night's sleep I'd be forever grateful."

January 13, 1931, age 48:
"Went to the doctor and got medicine for my sleeplessness." (I wonder what the "medicine" was.)

August 1, 1922, age 39:
"Put in a hard night, sleepless and worried."

About night sweats or hot flashes:

October 9, 1930, age 47:
"Slept with the window open last night. George [my grandfather] about froze, I was comfortable."

About difficulty concentrating:

February 17, 1929, age 46:
"My mind is not working lately."

About her changes in the mirror:

March 26, 1929, age 46:
"My dresses feel too tight around my middle."

May 4, 1929, age 46:
"Going to have to do something about my weight."

May 23, 1923, age 40:
"My skin is looking so dry. I must be getting old!"

About bladder or urinary symptoms:

August 20, 1923, age 40:
"Having problems with my bladder. Saw the doctor and he gave me some medicine."

About irregular periods:

January 13, 1931, age 48:
"Worried, could I be in a family way? I'm so late. I must get to the doctor." (The word *pregnant* was too indelicate for my grandmother.)

About changing energy patterns:

August 20, 1926, age 43:
"Canned 25 quarts of tomatoes. Spent the last part of the afternoon walking back to the woods, down the lane."

July 6, 1925, age 42:
"Should have hoed my garden today. Too tired. I picked some daisies instead."

About her changing role as a mother:

November 6, 1923, age 41:
"Maud brought over her niece. She's only two weeks old. What a beautiful baby. I thought of my own."

About the fact that she, and apparently her doctor, were uncertain as to the reasons for her physical and emotional symptoms:

September 24, 1924, age 41:
"I sure don't feel very well. Not sure what is wrong. The doctor says I'm fine."

October 10, 1924, age 42:
"Went to the doctor and had a rough time." (This was my grandmother's 42nd birthday. Now here I am speculating. The "rough

time" could refer to a painful exam, but I can't help but wonder if my grandmother tried to explain her tearfulness, changing periods, or other symptoms to her doctor, only to be told again that she was "fine.")

About giving and receiving in a community of women:

July 9, 1924, age 41:
"Need to spend more time at the church socials. Maud and I have such a good time."

July 23, 1930, age 47:
"Marianne's daughter died last night. She found her in her crib. All of the women from the church will go to her this afternoon."

Rereading my grandmother's journals with an eye toward how she may have felt during her forties was a tender and meaningful experience for me. I felt sad about her going through these changes alone, but I was also comforted and reassured to recognize that some of my own perimenopausal experiences parallel those she recorded over sixty years ago. It was inspiring to realize that she lived her life to the fullest for four more decades after perimenopause, working hard, caring about those she loved, making her mark on all of our lives, and demonstrating the kind of strength I believe is unique to women.

YOUR STORY

I first decided to ask for help when:

My first experience at the doctor's office was:

My doctor's appointment cost $_____ on _____ (date).

I chose my health care practitioner because:

(Family doctor? Recommended by a friend? Part of your insurance
    plan?)

When I left the doctor's office, I realized that:

(Did you feel like you had found the right place? Were you frustrated?
    Did you know that you had to search further?)

My physical symptoms were:

My emotional symptoms were:

I did/did not realize there was a connection between my physical and
emotional symptoms:

My interaction with my children was affected in the following ways:

I tried these alternative or complementary remedies:

My reasons for seeking alternative or complementary remedies were:

I was too embarrassed to ask questions about:

I did/did not belong to a support group:

My main concerns about family dynamics were:

My job concerns were:

My job has been affected by the changes I've experienced in these
ways:

If I put myself in my husband's shoes, I think he had these concerns
about me:

I think he had these concerns about his own aging:

If my intimate relationships have changed in my forties, this is an
example of how they are different:

When I think about my weight, these words come to mind:

The type of clothes I like to wear now are:

These clothes are (different from, similar to) clothes I was wearing ten
years ago:

Today when I look in the mirror at my skin, I most notice:

When I comb my hair, it looks:

My energy level is:

When my doctor talked with me about HRT, this is what she said:

My thoughts about HRT are:

The most confusing things to me about this period in my life are:

When these feelings of confusion are strong, I tend to react by:

I feel physically healthiest when:

I remember feeling especially effective and powerful when:

I have fun or spend a good time when I:

If only I had known _____ about what my forties would be like so far, here's what I would have done:

The person I talk to most about my physical and emotional changes is:

The person who provides me with the most understanding and support is:

The person who shows less understanding than I would like is:

The women (friends, family, or women in public life) I most admire are:

I admire these women because:

I exercise _____ per week.

My favorite form of exercise is:

The foods I eat most often are:

My daily caring rituals to make myself feel special include:

My greatest sources of inspiration and spiritual comfort are:

The times and places where I am most peaceful and centered are:

Date:

After writing your personal history, I suggest that you congratulate yourself for taking the time to do it. What did you learn about yourself? It's reinforcing to look over your reflections on aspects of your life that brought you contentment, satisfaction, and just plain *fun*. Make a conscious note of what you were doing at those times, where you were, and whom you were with, then include those people, places, and activities on all your "to do" lists. Sometimes we focus so much on where our trouble lies that we overlook our sources of help and encouragement.

Remember, you can always return to this section and add more so your personal history grows and changes along with you. You may choose to write the history as an exercise in introspection for yourself alone. Or if you do pass it along to family members, I guarantee they will share the delight and sentimentality I felt in rereading my grandmother's journal. Whether you keep your personal history simple and straightforward or detailed and elaborate, I hope you find that writing about changes during your forties develops and nourishes your inner life, where your wellspring of peace and strength lies.

Epilogue

Nurturing this book from the seed of an idea that came to me five years ago to the completion of the last chapter has, in many ways, mirrored and paralleled my own life transition during my forties. Through the inevitable fits and starts that are part of any creative project, I have continually reminded myself to practice what I preach and put what I've learned in eighteen years in the field of women's health into action: Learning from women I respect, personally and professionally. Adopting a flexible stance when an original concept didn't materialize. Taking a break and getting away when ideas seemed to languish. Starting all over, more than once, even when certain obstacles seemed insurmountable. Mining my own family history for inspiration, and finding it again in my grandmother's journals and in my memories of my grandfather's deep pleasure in and satisfaction with all of the stages of life.

This book progressed along with life's admixture of challenge, joy and pain. I made exciting changes in my women's health clinic to keep pace with technological and scientific developments. I saw one son joyfully married, grieved when his marriage ended, and prepared again to welcome a new family member when my younger son announced his engagement. My stepfather's sudden death seemed to eerily recall the loss of my father over two decades ago, reminding me once more to live in each moment, to slow the pace and breathe in all the reasons I am happy to be alive. When my mother's health necessitated her move into assisted living, I was grateful to have the opportunity to help her sift through a lifetime of her memories. In celebrating thirty years of marriage, my husband and I looked back with love and fondness and ahead with renewed devotion and commitment not only to growing older, but happier still, together.

As much as my professional role centers on helping women who need support and information about their hormonal health, the continual learning and growth I take from their examples brings a rich reciprocity to my experiences. Again and again, as I see forties women on their very individual journeys through physical, emotional, and spiritual changes, I hear about the value of our life experiences, the grace that comes with a deepening understanding of our own wisdom and power, and the need to let go of parts of our past, no matter how difficult, in order to move on. Media images notwithstanding, I see women who demonstrate the true definition of beauty in their happiness and their strength.

Not long before this book was complete, one of my patients, Gloria, added what I thought was a lovely grace note to the harmony of searching, wisdom, and answers that forties women have shared with me. If you recall, the first time she and I talked, she was impatient to get her perimenopausal changes over with, as if this part of her life were a nuisance she would just as soon dispense with. Since then she has done a lot of reading, reflecting, and talking with other women, and she more completely trusts the significance of her experiences and the power to be gained from them. When we talked a few weeks ago, Gloria said, "I realized I could let these years pool around me and stagnate if I didn't celebrate this point in my life, and recognize that this transition is mine both to learn and gather strength from." She told me she had developed a greater sense of serenity as her vision of herself in her forties had changed shape and become more complete.

After my chance meeting with Gloria (we ran into each other at a bookstore), it struck me that her conscious choice to embrace her changes, and the difference I saw in her face and demeanor, resulted from a fundamental and innate process of moving from struggle to resolution. The questions we ask and the truth revealed to us in our forties come from the same place: our powerful intuition, our connectedness to our own spirits, and the sage and perceptive messages spoken in the gentle language of our own hearts.

PERIMENOPAUSE: WHAT MEN WANT TO KNOW

When I mentioned to friends and colleagues that I wanted to include a section on men in my book on perimenopause, I got reactions ranging from an enthusiastic "Of course" to a blunt "Why in the world?" My conversations with forties women and the men who care about them led me to conclude that the book wouldn't be complete without a discussion of how our perimenopausal changes appear to and affect the men in our lives. In discussions with men, I realized that in facing age-related changes, they rarely mention their conflicting feelings about growing older. Most of all, they were unclear about perimenopause — what it is, what changes accompany it, and how they could best support the women for whom they care deeply while it is going on.

There has been little enough support and information about the perimenopausal transition geared toward women; I can't imagine where men would get information about this process. In this chapter, we'll take a look at questions men who are husbands or partners of women I see at my clinic frequently ask:

+ What happens physiologically during perimenopause?
+ Is perimenopause the same as menopause? As PMS?
+ How do hormones affect my partner's moods?
+ How long does perimenopause last?
+ Can I expect it to get better with time?
+ Is there something she can take that will help?
+ What can I do to help?

Many men ask me for strategies to help their wives, as Janice's husband, John, did. Some of Janice's escalating anxiety may have been hormonal, but in large part it had been recently heightened by her concern about her aging mother, her stepson's acting-out behavior, and the tension this created with John. John wanted to know how he could help

Janice without getting on her nerves, since she seemed so tense and edgy that anything he said or suggested rubbed her the wrong way. Other men have asked me: "What do I do if she bursts into tears over something trivial?" "How can I help her not to be so worried and anxious about everything?" "What do we say to the kids to help them understand what's going on?" I'll outline some of the specific steps men and women have told me were helpful in understanding each other and in opening up an honest dialogue.

If your partner in life is a perimenopausal woman, these are the things I hope will click in your mind and help make more sense of this transition. To begin, I'd like you to realize that you shouldn't expect to comprehend all the nuances of perimenopause. No one does yet, and every woman experiences it with her own unique style. I don't think there's a way to fully appreciate what it's like to be suddenly flushed and sweaty from a hot flash when you're trying to make an important presentation, or to have runaway feelings of anxiety that are disproportionate to anything going on in your life.

The information in the next pages will, however, help you see that without enough information, perimenopausal changes can seem confusing, frightening, annoying, or all three. What you can expect to have is a broad understanding of what your partner is going through. With understanding and support, the perimenopausal transition actually empowers and frees women to realize and appreciate the fullness of their experiences and wisdom. Finally, my intention is also to help you gain insight into your own feelings about aging, and to open the door to talk more about shared concerns. Understanding and discussing each other's changing life issues with honesty and concern brings comfort and strength to a relationship that may itself be in transition.

A DECADE OF SHARED CHANGE

The decade between ages 40 and 50 brings changes for women *and* men—some of them tumultuous, some more easily and calmly accepted. But among the forties couples I've met with and interviewed for this book, one thing stands out: these changes in our bodies, our sexuality, and in the way we view our life goals very rarely get talked about or even openly acknowledged among men and women. If they're discussed at all, the focus tends to be on what is happening with the woman.

When Mary's mood swings spilled over into her relationship with her fiancé, Ted, he tended to see what he called her "irrational irritability" as the root of the problems between them. Mary would defensively shoot back, "What would you blame our problems on if it weren't for my hormones?" At one point, when the cycle of quarreling and estrangement made both of them feel they had reached their limit, they considered canceling their wedding.

Men and women in their forties have more in common than they usually realize. Their bodies are changing, their sex life may be different, and they often review their direction and accomplishments during this time. While two people's lives are changing, many times they can't seem to fall in step, even when they privately long to lean on each other for support.

Why is this? For one thing, little attention has been given to how people change in their forties, because aside from the usual hoopla on a fortieth birthday, the decade itself isn't known for its milestones. Yet we're learning more and more about the changes women experience in this time, and how these changes affect their lives and, yes, their relationships. Rather than isolating this transition as strictly female and largely hormonal, let's view the forties decade as a time of joint transformation, one where thoughtful discussion of our respective needs builds our understanding of each other and of ourselves.

In essence, you and your partner are both going through one more life development together, adjusting to physical, emotional, and external changes. You've done this before: when you were first married and had to get used to sharing a bathroom, mingling your finances, and participating in a new set of family traditions, among other major adjustments and compromises. There may have been years when one of you concentrated heavily on advancing your career, and you both patterned your schedules in such a way to support that goal. If you have had a family, you'll remember what it was like to adapt to life as parents, trading nights out for time at home with the kids and learning to tread carefully over toys on the floor. Now you're witnessing the changes your partner is going through, while you wrestle with some of your own.

Usually "male menopause" is the stuff of lame jokes. But if we use the term to refer to the physical and emotional changes that occur in men at midlife, then yes, men do experience certain changes. Certainly male and female physiology are very different, but people of both genders in their forties often have parallel concerns, not only about their appearance and health but sometimes even about our larger spiritual purpose in life.

It may seem like only yesterday that you were entirely secure and confident about your body—youthful invincibility meant you rarely even *thought* about your health. But maybe now as you read the newspaper, you find your eyes stealing over to the ads. A local hospital offers prostate cancer screening. Should you go? you wonder. Or perhaps you find yourself worrying about your family history, as Daniel did. "My dad had a heart attack at fifty-two," he told me. "That's only five years older than I am now." Or maybe you still think health concerns are for "older" men, a word that won't apply to *you* for several more decades.

Even if you don't worry about your cholesterol or when you're due for a prostate exam, you may be concerned about visible changes in your body. The solid build you once had may be different now, and while you can't pinpoint exactly when it changed, it looks as if gravity has done some work. "My major issue is weight," said Alan. "I seem to study my body daily for weight gain and loss, and I always want to be slimmer." And those gray hairs—not only on your head but on your chest and elsewhere. How did they get there all of a sudden? It took a photograph to make Keith realize his appearance had changed. "I see myself every day in the mirror," he admitted. "But when I saw an old snapshot, it hit me that, wow, my hair and mustache used to be brown. Now they're pretty snowy."

Steve, Sharon's husband, had a brush with a life-threatening illness at 48, providing an unexpected view of his own mortality that left him badly shaken and somehow chastened in a way he couldn't fully describe. Worried about his own health and feeling guilty about the strain Sharon was under, Steve described himself as "completely unprepared" for the abrupt reversal in his previously good health. It's not uncommon for men and women in our age group to know someone— a sibling, friend, or co-worker—who develops a serious health problem.

This sobering experience gives us pause and sometimes prompts a reevaluation of what we are doing and why.

Along with noticing, or not noticing as the case may be, physical changes, maybe you're also mulling over other effects of the march of time. In the workplace there are both advantages and liabilities to being older and more experienced. You may have heard about or experienced a situation where a younger person rose faster in the competitive workplace, charging ahead with advanced computer skills, willing to work for less money and fewer benefits, and showing an aggressive edge that made you feel dull in comparison. The pressure escalates, and we worry about keeping up.

While this is going on in your own life, you've probably observed changes in your wife or partner. In perimenopause, she may look or act very different, or even seem like a different person from the woman you fell in love with and married. I'll explain these changes and offer recommendations on ways you can best support her during this transition.

Let's define *perimenopause*. First, it's neither an illness nor a signal that something is wrong with your partner. It's a period of approximately seven to ten years, during which the female reproductive system gradually slows down. Usually this occurs when women are between 40 and 50, although some women begin experiencing perimenopausal changes in their mid- to late thirties.

Here's what happens when a woman is in perimenopause:

+ Her estrogen levels gradually drop. In her fully fertile, reproductive years, her estrogen levels likely ranged from 0.5 to 5.0 pg/ml (when measured with a saliva sample). By the time she is fully menopausal and has stopped menstruating, these levels may range from 0.5 to 1.5 pg/ml.

+ The effects of her decline in estrogen may include:
hot flashes and/or night sweats
vaginal dryness that makes intercourse difficult
changes in mood and memory
reduced sex drive

thinning of the bones

urine leaks

increased risk of heart disease

+ As estrogen levels become lower, other hormone levels also dwindle, including those of progesterone and testosterone.

+ Estrogen and other hormones do not necessarily decline steadily during perimenopause. They may fluctuate, rising and falling at unpredictable times.

We don't know everything yet about how and why female hormones influence women's mood and memory. We do understand that there is a relationship between these hormones and some chemicals produced in the brain such as serotonin, dopamine, and norepinephrine. Sometimes these substances are called "feel good" chemicals. Without estrogen's nourishing effects, it's believed that brain levels of these important chemicals drop, which may produce bouts of depression, irritability, or tears. Such mood changes can often seem unpredictable and unrelated to any external cause. In addition, the calming effect of the reproductive hormone progesterone may no longer be present during perimenopause, so that an occasional tension seems to become unremitting anxiety.

Memory changes can also result from estrogen fluctuations. If your partner seems to be forgetful or says she has trouble concentrating, there is a possible hormonal explanation for it, although it's certainly not the only one. Estrogen's relationship with the brain chemical acetylcholine, which helps us call up information we've stored in our brains, may be imbalanced during perimenopause. But forgetfulness can also signal that the person has too much to do and too many details to manage without enough help. When a woman who prides herself on being detailed and organized comes to me because she has started to have trouble recalling things or keeping details straight in her mind, I generally evaluate the possible hormonal component of this change. I also review her daily agenda with her to see where she can delegate and ask for help. If your partner turns to you for some extra assistance, there are three things I suggest:

- Remember that it may not be easy for her to ask for help, especially with something she has previously handled with ease.
- Recognize that in asking you, she is singling you out as the person she relies on and trusts.
- If your own schedule is chock full, resist the temptation to look for reasons why the tasks or chores your partner has asked for help with don't need to be done. Instead, take a look at what you also might let go or delegate (not to your partner) in order to free some time.

JOINT (AND BONE) EXERCISE

Estrogen also acts as a kind of shoehorn, if you will, influencing the absorption of calcium by the bones. Women with lowered estrogen levels are at higher risk of osteoporosis, or thinning of the bones. Often osteoporosis exhibits no symptoms until a brittle bone fractures. In addition to calcium and vitamin D supplementation, regular weight-bearing exercise is the simplest and best form of insurance against osteoporosis. Men can develop osteoporosis too, although the incidence among women is higher.

I often recommend that couples exercise together, both as a means of protecting their bones and hearts, reducing stress, and as a healthy way of spending time together. It can take some creativity to combine two busy schedules, so I frequently suggest starting out by walking together once or twice a week — early morning or twilight are pleasant times to be together, and the extra endorphins will either start or end your day with a sense of well-being. Walking is also noncompetitive, costs nothing, and needs no equipment other than comfortable shoes. Don't be deceived by the fact that walking sounds tediously simple. I encounter many couples who agree to walk together only grudgingly but later tell me they have their "best talks" when they are out looking at morning's promise or dusk's lengthening shadows.

If you wish, choose a variety of ways to exercise together that suit both of your lifestyles and personalities:

- A joint membership at a gym doesn't necessarily have to mean pumping the machines together. Swimming is a great way to relax and condition your bodies. It doesn't take the place of the weight-bearing exercise your bones need, but it's a pleasant way to alternate an exercise routine.

✦ Try a new way to exercise your bodies together. If neither of you is familiar with yoga or tai chi, you may enjoy taking a class as a couple. Joint lessons can also be fun, be they in golf or tennis or in horseback riding or canoeing. Pick a sport or activity that you will both enjoy improving or learning for the first time.

✦ Dancing is wonderful exercise. You can move the furniture to make an impromptu dance floor at home and turn on your favorite music or plan an evening at a club. If you tend to groan when you're pulled to your feet at a wedding or bar mitzvah, think about taking a class together, and have fun with whatever form you choose. Line, ballroom, and swing are just a few possibilities.

MATTERS OF THE HEART

When the body's production of estrogen slows down, the likelihood of heart disease, the number-one cause of death among women, increases. That's because estrogen prevents the buildup of plaque on artery and vein walls. Without this protective effect, clogged arteries can result. Estrogen also helps to stabilize cholesterol levels, another benefit that declines in perimenopause. Some lifestyle patterns can build cardiovascular strength—for example, a diet that is low in fat and that includes holistic combinations of foods with soy protein and omega-3 fatty acids, a concerted effort to reduce stress, and a program of regular exercise.

You can join your partner in guarding against heart disease not only by exercising together but by sharing in her willingness to experiment with new foods and by supporting her as she claims time for herself to decompress and restore her energy. Take a moment to think about some of the perhaps silent and unseen things your partner does that are a regular part of making your family life work—shopping, cooking, doing laundry, transporting children, making doctor and dentist appointments, keeping the house organized, taking care of finances, and remembering anniversaries, birthdays, bar and bat mitzvahs, and graduations. I'm not suggesting that your partner, or women in general for that matter, always take full responsibility for these things, but if anything comes to mind that you could volunteer to do to give her a block of time for herself, I guarantee that she will be surprised, delighted, and grateful.

Many women tell me that an afternoon or evening in which they could do as they pleased would be a rare and very precious gift. There are several ways you can arrange to give this treat to your spouse:

+ If your wife would enjoy being home alone for a few hours, you can make the evening really special for her. Arrange to have a housekeeping crew come early in the morning, then take yourself and the family out for the rest of the day, leaving her at home. She'll love the peacefulness of a quiet, spotless house.

+ If time away from home is a pleasure for her, plan in advance for her to take an entire day without any responsibility for chores or errands. She'll love the opportunity to visit friends, hike, browse in shops, or do whatever feels like "time off" for her.

+ On a busy weekday, bring home takeout dinner and a magazine, book, or video that your wife will like. Many women I know find it hard to relax in the evening during the week—they catch up on a variety of work or family-related tasks. You may need to gently insist that she sit down, put her feet up, and take time to read or watch a movie for an evening, while you take over whatever needs to be done.

CHANGES IN THE MIRROR

The symptoms of perimenopause cover a vast territory—they go way beyond an occasional hot flash. A woman's hormones affect her looks too, and when perimenopausal physical changes start to occur, a woman's self-esteem, her perception of herself, and even her view of her relationship with you can undergo some seismic transformations.

As women get older, their basal metabolic rate changes, which means that they need fewer calories to maintain the same weight. Not all perimenopausal women gain weight, but some find that no matter how closely they watch what they eat, they grow softer and rounder in their forties. A woman who weighed 125 and who averaged 2,200 calories daily for years may well see her body shape change, to become more generous in the hips, thighs, and abdomen, and straighter in the waist, if she eats the same way in her forties. Before Alan understood that the differences in his wife's body were connected to changes in her metabolism, he wondered if she was getting "heavier" or "forgetting to take care of herself."

I explained that in all likelihood, neither was true. As a woman's ovarian function declines, her body continues to produce estrogen, but a different type of estrogen and in smaller amounts. As her ovaries become less active, her fat cells play a key role in synthesizing estrogen, so the change in body shape is actually part of nature's protectiveness.

Hormonally influenced weight or body changes can be accompanied by other changes in appearance if a woman hasn't taken the time she needs to eat well or rest herself physically and mentally. Chemical shifts in the body don't have to take their toll on women's skin and hair. Women can help to minimize the facial lines, dry skin, and lusterless hair that sometimes result from estrogen loss not only with herbs, diet, and exercise but also by seeking out sources of inspiration and joy through their work, friends, and relationships. Happiness is beauty in the forties.

Sometimes men make what they think is an innocent or merely observational comment about something different about their wife or partner's appearance, only to be met with a storm of anger or tears, a frosty silence, or an expression of deep hurt. Rather than comment on a physical change, here are some specific actions you can take that will remind your partner that you cherish her inside and out:

+ Put a photo of her in a prominent place. You can frame one from your collection, put a favorite one into a brand-new, special frame, or if she would enjoy having a new picture taken, arrange a date and time for the session. Let her know that you like to look at her picture and think about all she means to you.

+ Plan a day trip to a spa where you can both enjoy hot springs, a steam bath, a massage, a facial, or other body and soul-nurturing pleasures. You will both feel invigorated, relaxed, and renewed afterward.

+ Invite your partner to an evening out where there will be a crowd — a popular restaurant, a concert, a sold-out play. Tell her your express purpose is to show the masses that she is the loveliest and most important person in your life.

THE MOOD OF THE FORTIES

Every woman responds to perimenopausal changes differently, depending on her personality. Some become withdrawn and remote, like Alan's wife. "She was depressed and detached," he said. "It was confusing. I found it hard to tell how much of the aloofness was due to me, something I was doing, or how much was externally caused. I also wondered if maybe her personality had just changed." Other women show more aggression, hostility, or irritability during perimenopause. For still others, if they don't fully understand what their bodies, minds, and spirits are going through, the changes have a confusing, frightening or almost paralyzing effect.

It's only recently that medical professionals have started to pay closer attention to perimenopausal changes, most likely because women of the baby boom generation have learned to insist upon and expect better health care. In fact, the term *perimenopause* only recently came into being. Still, the shortage of information about what women can expect during their forties is still acute, and even less has been written or discussed that would give those intimately involved with them any understanding of what to do or how to act when mood changes bring unforeseen elements into a relationship.

Just as some women are bewildered by changes in the way they look and feel, some men aren't quite sure how to handle perimenopause's unpredictable effects. "I had finally figured out how my wife's menstrual cycle affected her mood. I knew when to expect irritability and tears at times. We had worked out that I needed to stay out of her way and that she shouldn't take anything I said personally during that time." This was from Dave, whose wife, Lisa, is now perimenopausal and whose menstrual cycle is no longer like clockwork. "Now I have no idea what to expect, or when. The predictability factor is gone," he said.

Dave said he felt helpless and confused. He genuinely wanted to know what he could do to help Lisa, but wasn't sure where to start. "Last week we had to change our vacation schedule because of my work. She broke down in tears. I didn't think she would take it so hard—it seemed like a trivial thing to me." These storms of tears were happening more and more frequently, Dave said.

"Try making a simple show of interest and support," I suggested. "When something is upsetting Lisa, you might begin by putting an arm around her shoulders. Let her know you're willing to put your heads together and figure out how to make something work, or how to change something that is bothering her." I assured Dave that this gesture would probably be met with gratitude and relief. He agreed to try it the next time Lisa was upset. I also gently observed that what seemed trivial to Dave clearly was not trivial to Lisa, and that it was important to resist judging or dismissing her concerns.

Tears. Moodiness. A snappish, angry tone of voice. It can be tough not to react by getting angry yourself and telling your partner that whatever is bothering her is "no big deal." But demonstrating your support will give her the option of letting you know what she wants to do, and what help she needs from you. It also makes her feel less alone. Remember, though, that supporting her isn't the same as directing her. Even if you're an expert problem solver and even if you're convinced you have a perfect, easy solution to her particular dilemma, she probably isn't looking for anyone to tell her how to fix it.

If your partner seems especially irritable, depressed, or anxious, there are several ways you can help:

+ Avoid asking "What's wrong?" or "What did I do?" You may genuinely want to know, but many women have told me these questions are not helpful. In many cases, her feelings are not about you or anything you did.

+ Acknowledge her feelings without judging or blaming her. Sometimes a simple statement like "I can see that you're upset today— I'm here if you need me" can make a huge difference in the way she feels.

+ Make your offer to help as specific as you can. Some men tell me they ask their partners, "Is there anything I can do?" Take this generous gesture one step further by being precise: "I'd be glad to

take the kids out for dinner this evening so you can have a break."
"I'll buy, wrap, and mail Grandpa's birthday gift." "I'll get the groceries we need."

SEXUALITY IN THE FORTIES

During perimenopause, the experience of sexual intimacy can change, partly in response to hormonal fluctuations. The female genitourinary tract depends on estrogen to be healthy, so the bladder, urethra, external genitalia, and vaginal canal are all affected by declining estrogen levels. If it seems to you that your partner has become less passionate, or even plain uninterested in making love or unresponsive when you want to, avoid making assumptions about why this is happening. It doesn't necessarily mean that she is less attracted to you, or that she cares more about the kids or her job than you. For one thing, hormonal changes in some perimenopausal women cause a vaginal dryness that makes intercourse uncomfortable or even painful. Getting a lubricant can help, as can slowing down or finding other ways to touch and show love besides intercourse. A waning sex drive can also be due to shifting hormone levels—her body is making less testosterone, the hormone that sparks sexual desire. Women who become depressed during perimenopause often say they are less interested in sex.

There's also another possible reason for a drop in sexual desire: your partner may just be too tired to want to make love. Many perimenopausal women have trouble sleeping—their sleep may be restless and fragmented. Researchers are now taking a closer look at how estrogen regulates brain chemicals that play an important role in inducing sleep. Night sweats, also resulting from hormonal surges, may also be keeping her tossing and turning at night, waking up feeling like she hasn't slept at all.

Both the emotional and physical ease of lovemaking may be changing for you as well. At the same time your partner is experiencing hormonal fluctuations, your own sexual response may be changing. Some forties men find that it takes longer to achieve an erection, or that it is more difficult to maintain one. I recommended that both Alan and Dave talk with their wives about their concerns, fears, and suggestions.

Alan was concerned and admittedly angry at Susan about her aloofness and for what he mistakenly thought was her lack of care for her physical appearance. Dave wanted to know how best to respond to Lisa's seemingly mercurial mood changes. Yet neither of them had talked directly with their wives about these issues.

It may be that you, like Alan and Dave, haven't discussed your relationship with your partner for some time. If so, take time to share your concerns. You might want to suggest that you both make a list of issues to discuss, which may include:

- ✦ how you communicate and respond to each other in your day-to-day life together
- ✦ how you share responsibilities (household, financial, children)
- ✦ how you express passion and love

You can assemble your list of concerns in any way that works for you, whether by keeping notes in a calendar, in a notebook, or on the odd scrap of paper. If you're not inclined to write things down, make sure you take enough time to think carefully about your concerns and crystallize them in your mind. It may help to write or think about aspects of yourself that:

- ✦ confuse you
- ✦ are important to you
- ✦ you'd like to change

The best time to raise the suggestion that you and your partner review your concerns will be when you are both relaxed and doing something you enjoy, such as taking a walk or having dinner together. Set a time to discuss these concerns without interruptions from the rest of the family or the telephone. You may decide to talk over the issues that seem most important to you first and get to other concerns at another time — everything doesn't have to be ironed out or solved in one conversation. Instead, use the time you spend with your partner to gather and share information, and to let her know not only how much you care about her but that you are very invested in the relationship and want her to be as well.

Both Alan and Dave said the conversations they had with their wives gave them the chance to talk freely about their wives' perimenopausal changes as well as their feelings about their own aging. Without this chance, both Alan and Dave could have ended up feeling that all their time, energy, and attention were being devoted to attending to their wives' life changes, at the expense of their own. "Susan and I made some agreements about taking better care of our health," Alan said, "watching our weight and taking a walk together at least twice a week. We even made a date to spend one evening a week cooking a healthy meal together." His list of concerns also clued him in to something about himself: "I was upset with myself about the weight I've gained recently, and for not keeping in shape. It was easier to pay attention to Susan's weight than my own."

Dave agreed to play a part in getting at the root of Lisa's mood swings. "I'm going to go with her when she sees her doctor to talk about how teary and depressed she's been," he said. "Up until now I think she had been hesitant to go, but after we talked, she seemed glad that I volunteered to go with her. She said it felt supportive."

Mary's fiancé, Ted, simply said, "I had no idea," after he and I talked through some of the physiology of perimenopause and how it can affect the way women think, act, and feel. "It never occurred to me to think in terms of a physical transition," he told me. "I just assumed our relationship wasn't working anymore."

One day as I was in the middle of writing this part of the book, I tore off a new page on my daily calendar and found this saying: "Relationships don't need to be worked on, they need to be participated in." I thought it was a good reminder for men *and* women: neither of us is involved in a spectator sport here. As we move through our forties, we have choices about this transition as we do with all of life's passages and stages. It's sometimes tempting to resist change because we see it as a form of upheaval, but the perimenopausal transition can represent an opportunity for you and your partner to build a shared commitment to better health for both of you, and to breathe new life into your relationship in energizing and affirming ways.

RESOURCES

SALIVA HORMONE TESTING

Aeron LifeCycles
1933 Davis Street, Suite 310
San Leandro, CA 94577
(800) 631-7900

Madison Pharmacy Associates
429 Gammon Place
P.O. Box 259690
Madison, WI 53725
(800) 558-7046

NATURAL HORMONE REPLACEMENT THERAPY

Full Circle Women's Health
1800 30th Street, Suite 308
Boulder, CO 80301
(800) 418-4040
e-mail: womenshealth@hotmail.com
Web site: http://www.menopause-pms.com

Madison Pharmacy Associates
429 Gammon Place
P.O. Box 259690
Madison, WI 53725
(800) 558-7046
Web site:
http://www.womenshealth.com

PHYSICIAN REFERRAL

North American Menopause Society
University Hospitals
Department of Ob/Gyn
2074 Abington Road
Cleveland, OH 44016
(216) 844-8748

INFORMATION ON NATUROPATHY, HERBAL MEDICINE, AND HOMEOPATHY

American Association of Naturopathic Physicians
2366 Eastlake Avenue, Suite 322
Seattle, WA 98102
(206) 298-0125

American Botanical Council
P.O. Box 201660
Austin, TX 78720
Web site: http://www.herbalgram.org

Celestial Seasonings
4600 Sleepytime Drive
Boulder, CO 80301-3292
(303) 530-5300

Herb Research Foundation
1007 Pearl Street, Suite 200
Boulder, CO 80302
(303) 449-2265
Web site: http://sunsite.unc.edu/herbs/hrfinfo.html

Lawrence Review of Natural Products
111 West Port Plaza, Suite 300
St. Louis, MO 63146-3098
(800) 223-0554

PhytoPharmica
P.O. Box 1745
Green Bay, WI 54305
(800) 533-2370

YOGA

American Yoga Association
513 South Orange Avenue
Sarasota, FL 34236-7598
(941) 953-5859
Web site: http://users.aol.com/
amyogaassn
(Send a SASE with $.55 postage for
guidelines on choosing a qualified yoga
instructor and catalog of instructional
books and tapes for home practice.)

ACUPUNCTURE

National Commission for the
Certification of Acupuncturists
1424 16th Street N.W., Suite 105
Washington, DC 20036
(202) 232-1404

ACUPRESSURE

Acupressure Institute
1533 Shattuck Avenue
Berkeley, CA 94709
(800) 442-2232
e-mail: gach@acupressure.com
Web site: http://www.healthy.net/
acupressure

APPENDIX C

SELECTED REFERENCES

CHAPTER 1: PERIMENOPAUSE: THE BIG PICTURE

Greer, G. *The Change*. New York: Ballantine, 1991.

Landau, C. *The Complete Book of Menopause*. New York: Grosset/Putnam, 1994.

Notelovitz, M., and D. Tonnessen. *Menopause and Midlife Health*. New York: St. Martin's, 1993.

Sheehy, G. *The Silent Passage*. New York: Random House, 1991.

Wilson, R. A. *Feminine Forever*. New York: Evans, 1966.

CHAPTER 2: WHERE ARE YOU IN THE PROCESS?

Dalton, K. *The Premenstrual Syndrome and Progesterone Therapy*. Chicago: Yearbook Medical Publishers, 1977.

Bender, S., and K. Kelleher. *Premenstrual Syndrome: Women Tell Women How to Control PMS*. New York: New Harbinger, 1996.

Follingstad, A. H. "Estriol, the Forgotten Estrogen?" *Journal of the American Medical Association*, vol. 239 (1978), pp. 29–30.

Kleijnen, J., and P. Knipschild. "Ginkgo Biloba for Cerebral Insufficiency." *Lancet*, vol. 34 (1992) pp. 352–58.

Mindell, E. *Earl Mindell's Soy Miracle*. New York: Fireside, 1995.

Murray, M. T. "Remifemin: Answers to Some Common Questions." *American Journal of Natural Medicine*, vol. 4, no. 3 (1997), pp. 3–5.

Vliet, E. L. *Screaming to Be Heard: Hormonal Connections Women Suspect and Doctors Ignore*. New York: M. Evans and Co., 1995.

Women's Health America, Madison, Wisconsin. "Perimenopause to Menopause: A Positive Change of Life." 1997.

CHAPTER 3: THE HORMONAL LANDSCAPE

Dalton, K. *Once a Month*. Claremont, CA: Hunter House, 1990.

Ellison, P., et al. "Measurements of Salivary Progesterone." *Annals of the New York Academy of Science*, vol. 694 (1993), pp. 161–76.

Maxon, W. S. "Bioavailability of Oral Micronized Progesterone." *Fertility and Sterility*, vol. 44 (1985), pp. 121–28.

Regelson, W. *The Super-Hormone Promise*. New York: Simon and Schuster, 1996.

Vining, R. F., et al. "The Measurements of Hormones in Saliva: Possibilities and Pitfalls." *Journal of Steroid Biochemistry* vol. 27 (1987), pp. 81–94.

Vliet, E. L. *Screaming to Be Heard: Hormonal Connections Women Suspect and Doctors Ignore*. New York: M. Evans and Co., 1995.

Women's Health America, Madison, Wisconsin. "Perimenopause to Menopause: A Positive Change of Life." 1997.

CHAPTER 4: MEMORY, MOODS, AND PRODUCTIVITY

Henderson, V. W. "The Epidemiology of Estrogen Replacement Therapy and Alzheimer's Disease." *Neurology* vol. 48 (1997) pp. S27–S35.

Pierpaoli, W., et al. *The Melatonin Miracle*. New York: Simon and Schuster, 1995.

Sherwin, B., and L. Kampen. "Estrogen Use and Verbal Memory in Healthy Postmenopausal Women." *Obstetrics and Gynecology*, vol. 83, no. 6 (1994), pp. 979–83.

Tang, M. "Effect of Estrogen During Menopause on Risk and Age at Onset of Alzheimer's Disease." *Lancet*, vol. 348 (1996), pp. 429–32.

Vliet, E. "New Insights on Hormones and Mood." *Menopause Management* (June/July 1993), pp. 140–46.

Women's Health America, Madison, Wisconsin. "Perimenopause to Menopause: A Positive Change of Life." 1997.

CHAPTER 5: PLANNING AHEAD FOR HEALTHY HEART, BONES, AND BREASTS

Bernstein, L., et al. "Physical Exercise and Reduced Risk of Breast Cancer in Young Women." *Journal of the American Cancer Institute*, vol. 86, no. 18 (1994), pp. 1403–8.

Bonnick, S. L. *The Osteoporosis Handbook*. Dallas: Taylor Publishing, 1997.

Bush, T. L. "The Epidemiology of Cardiovascular Disease in Postmenopausal Women." *Annals of New York Academy of Sciences*, vol. 592 (1990) pp. 263–71, discussion 334–345.

Colditz, G. A., et al. "The Use of Estrogens and Progestins and the Risk of Breast Cancer in Postmenopausal Women." *New England Journal of Medicine*, vol. 332 (1995), pp. 1589–93.

Lee, H. P., et al. "Dietary Effects on Breast Cancer Risk in Singapore." *Lancet*, vol. 337 (1991), pp. 1197–1200.

Legato, M., and C. Colman. *The Female Heart*. New York: Simon and Schuster, 1991.

Love, S. M. *Dr. Susan Love's Breast Book*. Reading, MA: Addison-Wesley, 1995.

Prior, J. C. "Progesterone as a Bone-trophic Hormone." *Endocrine Reviews*, vol. 11 (1990), pp. 386–98.

Stanford, J. L., et al. "Combined Estrogen and Progestin Hormone Replacement Therapy in Relation to Risk of Breast Cancer." *Journal of the American Medical Association*, vol. 274 (1995), pp. 37–142.

Thune, I., et al. "Physical Activity and the Risk of Breast Cancer." *New England Journal of Medicine*, vol. 336 (1997), pp. 1269–75.

Writing Group for the PEPI Trial. "Effects of Estrogen or Estrogen/Progestin Regimens on Heart Disease Risk Factors in Postmenopausal Women: The Postmenopausal Estrogen/Progestin Interventions (PEPI) Trial." *Journal of the American Medical Association*, vol. 272, no. 3 (1995), pp. 199–208.

CHAPTER 6: HORMONE REPLACEMENT THERAPY: FACTS ABOUT YOUR CHOICES

Colditz, G. A., et al. "The Use of Estrogens and Progestins and the Risk of Breast Cancer in Postmenopausal Women." *New England Journal of Medicine*, vol. 332 (1995), pp. 1589–93.

Follingstad, A. H. "Estriol, the Forgotten Estrogen?" *Journal of the American Medical Association*, vol. 239 (1978), pp. 29–30.

Grodstein, F. "Postmenopausal Hormone Therapy and Mortality." *New England Journal of Medicine*, vol. 336 (1997), pp. 1769–75.

Hargrove, J. T., et al. "Absorption of Oral Progesterone Is Influenced by Vehicle and Particle Size." *American Journal of Obstetrics and Gynecology*, vol. 61, no. 4 (1989), pp. 948–51.

Lee, J., and V. Hopkins. *What Your Doctor May Not Tell You About Menopause: The Breakthrough Book on Natural Progesterone.* New York: Warner, 1996.

Love, S. *Dr. Susan Love's Hormone Book.* New York: Random House, 1997.

Martorano, J. T., et al. "Differentiating Between Natural Progesterone and Synthetic Progestogens: Clinical Implications for Premenstrual Syndrome Management." *Comprehensive Therapy*, vol. 19 (1993), pp. 96–98.

Nachtigall, L. E. "Emerging Delivery Systems for Estrogen Replacement: Aspects of Transdermal and Oral Delivery." *American Journal of Obstetrics and Gynecology*, vol. 173 (1995), pp. 993–97.

Stanford, J. L., et al. "Combined Estrogen and Progestin Hormone Replacement Therapy in Relation to Risk of Breast Cancer." *Journal of the American Medical Association*, vol. 274 (1995), pp. 37–142.

Women's Health America, Madison, Wisconsin. "Perimenopause to Menopause: A Positive Change of Life." 1997.

Women's Health America, Madison, Wisconsin. "Natural Hormone Replacement Therapy." 1997.

CHAPTER 7: COMPLEMENTARY MEDICINE IN THE FORTIES

Brown, E., and L. Walker. *Menopause and Estrogen: Natural Alternatives to Hormone Replacement Therapy.* Berkeley, CA: Frog, 1996.

Laux, M., and C. Conrad. *Natural Woman, Natural Menopause.* New York: HarperCollins, 1997.

Lee, H. P., et al. "Dietary Effects on Breast Cancer Risk in Singapore." *Lancet,* vol. 337 (1991), pp. 1197–1200.

Morales, A. J., et al. "Effect of Replacement Dose of DHEA in Men and Women of Advancing Age." *Journal of Clinical Endocrinological Metabolism,* vol. 12 (1994), pp. 415–17.

Murray, M. T. *The Healing Power of Herbs.* Rocklin, CA: Prima, 1995.

Tyler, V. E. *Herbs of Choice.* New York: Pharmaceutical Products Press, 1994.

CHAPTER 8: A DECADE OF SELF-CARE

Adlercreutz, H., et al., "Urinary Excretion of Lignans and Isoflavonoid Phytoestrogen in Japanese Men and Women Consuming a Traditional Japanese Diet." *American Journal of Clinical Nutrition,* vol. 54 (1991) pp. 1093–100.

Anderson, J. W. "Meta Analysis of the Effects of Soy Protein Intake on Serum Lipids." *New England Journal of Medicine,* vol. 333 (1995), pp. 276–82.

Feskanich, D., et al. "Protein Consumption and Bone Fractures in Women." *American Journal of Epidemiology,* vol. 143, no. 5 (1996), pp. 472–79.

Kent, H. *Yoga Made Easy: A Personal Yoga Program That Will Transform Your Daily Life.* Allentown, PA: People's Medical Society, 1991.

Kirby, C. *The Art of Sensual Yoga: A Step-by-Step Guide for Couples.* New York: Plume, 1997.

McFarlane, S. *The Complete Book of T'ai Chi.* New York: DK Publishing, 1997.

Naomi, O., et al. "Evaluation of the Effect of Soybean Milk and Soybean Milk Peptide on Bone Metabolism in the Rate Model with Ovariectomized Osteoporosis." *Journal of Nutritional Sciences and Vitaminol,* vol. 40 (1994), pp. 201–11.

Shangold, M. "Exercise in the Menopausal Woman." *Obstetrics and Gynecology,* vol. 75 (1990), pp. 535–85.

Wang, C., et al. "Effects of Isoflavones, Flavinoids, and Lignans on Proliferation of Estrogen-Dependent and Independent Human Breast Cancer Cells." *Proceedings of the American Association for Cancer Research,* vol. 37 (1996), p. 277.

CHAPTER 9: CHANGES IN THE MIRROR

Bauer, C. *Acupressure for Everyone; Gentle Effective Relief for More Than 100 Common Ailments.* New York: Henry Holt, 1991.

Danese, M. D., et al. "Screening for Mild Thyroid Failure at the Periodic Health Examination." *Journal of the American Medical Association*, vol. 276 (1996), pp. 285–92.

Gach, M. R. *Acu-Face Lift Beauty Workbook*. Berkeley, CA: Acupressure Institute, 1994.

CHAPTER 10: SEXUALITY IN THE FORTIES

McKinlay, J. B., et al. "The Relative Contributions of Endocrine Changes and Social Circumstances to Depression in Mid-aged Women." *Journal of Health and Social Behavior* (1987), pp. 345–63.

Rako, S. *The Hormone of Desire*. New York: Harmony, 1996.

Vliet, E. "New Insights on Hormones and Mood." *Menopause Management* (June/July 1993), pp. 140–46.

Women's Health America, Madison, Wisconsin. "Perimenopause to Menopause: A Positive Change of Life." 1997.

Young, R. L. "Androgens in Postmenopausal Therapy?" *Menopause Management*, vol. 2, no. 5 (1993), pp. 21–24.

CHAPTER 11: EMPTY NEST/FULL NEST

Dalton, K. *Depression After Childbirth*. London: Oxford University Press, 1980.

Dix, C. *The New Mother Syndrome*. New York: Doubleday, 1985.

Doress, P. B., and D. L. Siegal. *Ourselves Growing Older*. New York: Simon and Schuster, 1987.

Podolsky, D. "Having Babies Past 40." *U.S. News & World Report* (October 29, 1990).

Sloan, G. *Postponing Parenthood*. New York: Plenum, 1993.

FSH (follicle-stimulating hormone), 4
  in menstrual cycle, 36
  normal levels, 46
  surges as cause of hot flashes, 6, 44, 54–55
  testing for levels, 44–45

genitourinary tract, 143–44, 193–94
  See also vaginal dryness
Germany, 126–27
ginkgo biloba, 21, 60, 139–40
ginseng, Siberian, 60, 145
goldenseal, 144

Hahnemann, Samuel, 147
hair, facial, 187–88
Harrison, Michelle, 33
headaches, 111, 144
heart, effects of estrogen, 73–74
heart disease
  benefits of hormone replacement therapy, 75
  reducing risk of, 77–78, 91, 92, 93, 120
  risk of, 73, 74
  symptoms, 75–76
  treatment of women, 76–77
herbal preparations, 122, 126–27
  aphrodisiacs, 144–45
  for headaches, 144
  for hot flashes, 22, 137, 141–43
  memory boosters, 21, 60, 139–40
  mood balancers, 130–37
  reliable sources, 129
  sedatives, 58, 134–35, 137
  selecting, 105
  for urinary tract infections, 144
herbs
  angelica, 142
  chamomile, 138
  chaste tree berry, 142
  damiana, 145
  false unicorn root, 145
  feverfew, 144
  ginkgo biloba, 21, 60, 139–40
  goldenseal, 144
  licorice, 142–43
  Siberian ginseng, 60, 145
  St. John's wort, 69, 135–37
  uva ursi, 144
  See also black cohosh
homeopathy, 146–48
hormone replacement therapy (HRT)
  adjusting dosages, 46–47, 117–18, 119

alternatives to, 97, 133–34
benefits for moods, 42–43, 64–65, 66–67, 109–10
brand names, 101–2
breast cancer and, 86, 114–15
candidates for, 28–29
components, 29, 102–4, 106–7, 109–10
cyclic or continuous, 113–14
decision to use, 119, 120–21
duration, 119–21
effects on breasts, 184
forms, 47, 101–2, 111–13, 117
hormone options, 100–102
location of application, 47
patient compliance, 108–9
physical benefits, 75, 81, 115, 120, 195–96
risks, 114–15
side effects, 107, 115–17, 120–21
testosterone, 29, 197–200
weight gain, 116–17
hormones, 32–34
  actions in brain, 7, 33, 41, 55
  bones and, 80
  DHEA, 140–41, 197
  intuition about changes, 49–50
  melatonin, 55–56, 138
  in menstrual cycle, 35–38, 39–40
  natural, 100, 104–5
  normal levels, 46
  sources, 105–6
  synthetic, 104–5
  testing, 43–47, 48–50
  thyroid, 8, 181–82
  See also estrogen; FSH; progesterone; testosterone
hot flashes, 40
  causes, 6, 44, 54–55
  palpitations accompanying, 76
  remedies, 22, 141–43
HRT. *See* hormone replacement therapy

infertility, 217–21
insomnia, 6–7, 54, 55–56, 202–3, 216
  remedies, 56–58, 137–38
intimacy, 208–10
  See also sexuality
intuition, about hormonal changes, 49–50
ipriflavone, 97
iron, 172
isoflavones, 25–26

journals. *See* personal histories